Anatomy for Runners

Unlocking Your Athletic Potential for
Health, Speed, and Injury Prevention

JAY DICHARRY, MPT, SCS

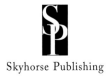

Skyhorse Publishing

Information presented in this book does not constitute medical advice. We recommend consulting with a qualified medical practitioner regarding any existing injuries and before making any changes to your training.

To my mom and dad for the lessons
To my wife for the love
To my kids for the future
To my friends for support
And to Ferris Bueller for daily inspiration
Thanks—Jay

Contents

Preface

A long time ago, there was a boy who swam. He trained about 15 to 18 hours a week in the water, counting pool tiles and singing in his head to pass the time. The high school cross-country coach was looking to recruit individuals for the team. The boy was recruited (OK—forced, it was private school) to run. This little lad wasn't really into the idea, but found he loved it. Instead of counting pool tiles, he could actually have a conversation while training. He could look up at the sky, feel the wind, and smell the fresh exhaust coming out of the tailpipe of each passing car (this was the city). Due to his swimming fitness, he made gains quickly. However, injuries were his biggest nemesis. He'd get hurt and need to take time off. After recovery he ran again, only to find the same pains. He went to expert orthopedists. These doctors told him that his "parts" were fine—they said to take some time off or (worse) stop running.

This answer didn't really sit well with him. His friends and teammates all ran much more than he did, and they weren't getting hurt. He was spending so many hours training his heart and lungs in the pool that it was practically a part-time job. Each and every day, he did tons of drills, repeats, and lifted weights to help him become a better swimmer. But in cross-country practice, all he had to do was run . . . and he kept getting hurt. And all the while the docs said his parts were fine and maybe they weren't working right together.

If you guessed that this boy was me, you'd be right. As long as we are coming clean here, I should let you know that the reason I entered health care was not to "help others" like everyone writes on their application essay. I wanted to get into health care because I got sick and tired of getting generic information. "Your X-ray is clean. Rest. Take time off." OK—I did all that and then tried to resume running, and it would come right back within a few weeks. My vicious cycle of running, injury, rest continued throughout my entire high school career. By the time I got to college, I was so sick of it, I stopped running for years. I couldn't find anyone who could look past my symptoms and get to the root of my problem.

A lot of you have been in my shoes (excuse the pun). Or maybe you coach or treat runners who always seem to fall into the same injury cycle that they just can't break. So this work is a summary of what I've learned over my personal, educational, and professional career. I am going to come at all of this from a different angle than most of what you've heard in the past because the realm I operate in combines the very different fields of clinical care, biomechanical analysis, and coaching.

The experts in these fields all have very different mind-sets. Clinicians use their brains to cluster your signs and symptoms to arrive at a diagnosis. In patient care, it's rare that things are 100 percent the same in 100 percent of the people, 100 percent of the time. Clinicians look for a variety of things to "line up." The advantage to this approach is that it guides your intervention to solve the current problem and makes you feel better at the present. This focus on symptoms masks the pain and makes it challenging to identify the root of the problem. Sometimes the cause is rather obvious, such as a sharp transition in training load, but often, there is a critical imbalance that shifts the repetitive overload on the body's tissues. If the body can't adapt, it breaks. Wouldn't identifying the imbalance help?

Scientists, namely biomechanists, are much more objective in nature. They are trying to find "the answer." Their contribution to the theory and foundation of running science has been, and continues to be, overwhelmingly positive. They ask questions, find answers, and come up with yet more questions. While this is intellectually stimulating, biomechainsts don't treat the individual patients and have no idea how to actually help *you*. People are by nature, variable. While it's tough to find the exact reasons why *groups* of people have certain injuries, or become efficient, or don't, it's even tougher to identify the reasons impacting each and every person *individually*. Getting "the answer" is very hard!

Coaches are results–focused. You, Mom, Dad, the team, the sponsors all want the big "W." Good coaches listen first. Guys and gals, I'll let you in on a little secret: There is no magical workout. The art of coaching is all about figuring out how your athletes will respond to your training plan and tailoring the timing of the program to their needs. Coaches are steadfast, honorable folks that we can look up to because they really do have our best interests at heart. They are trained to listen to your body and tailor the workout dose and timing to you. But when we start asking why a runner got a stress fracture or what shoes they should be in or how to return a runner following their injury, we realize that these folks typically lack the knowledge and resources to answer the questions that face them. It's outside of their job description.

I'd like to share a quote from a physician named Tom Novacheck: "Much can be gained if the biomechanist and pathophysiologist come out of the laboratory, the clinician pulls himself out of the clinic, and they all meet on the track." All parties bring critical information to get to the root of the issue. If you approach running by combining the theory of movement, a thorough understanding of the individual's strengths and weaknesses, and training loads, you begin to find answers. This is what I've tried to do in my career as a clinician, coach, and researcher, and what I've tried to do for you in this book.

While we (as a scientific and clinical community) don't have all the answers to every risk factor of every injury, we do know a lot. The media is encouraged to focus on the latest trends and *the one exercise every runner must do this fall!* This book's aim is to reveal how the musculoskeletal system responds to running and how to optimize this relationship. I'd like to help you help yourself. Read it for your own knowledge. Read it to help the kids you coach. Read it to prep yourself for the next visit to your trusted health care provider about a running injury. Clinicians will even find this book closes the loopholes in applying their knowledge to runners. Knowledge is power, and all that rah-rah stuff. Think of it as Volume 2 of *Inside Your Outside* by Dr. Seuss (not required reading, but highly recommended). So together, we'll embark on a mission to tackle two main points:

1. **Anatomy:** What are your parts and what is unique about them? And how does running affect them?
2. **The Athlete Within:** Learn how to optimize the function of your parts to combat injury risk and improve performance with specific exercise prescriptions and form tips.

In answering those two points, this book focuses on three areas:

1. **Theory:** Each and every time I present, someone comes up to me and asks, "Where can I find more resources about what you do?" To be honest, there aren't really any "approachable" biomechanics texts out there. And there aren't really any "approachable" clinical books out there either. So one of the main drives of this project was to bestow some critical knowledge about biomechanics and how the body responds to training. Let's be honest, this first section is not summer beach reading. But if you *really* want to know *why* your parts are different and *how* those differences play out, give it a read. It's like worrying about meeting your girlfriend's parents for the first time. Yes, it's scary, but you have to come to terms with it because it's not going away. This foundation impacts every other thing in this book.

2. **Applied:** So your body's parts don't just live in a display case in a museum; they interact as you run, they require a certain amount of motion and a certain amount of stability. The technique with which you run also plays a critical role. We'll explore how running influences the body and how the body influences your running.

3. **Interventional:** Hopefully, after reading this book through, you are feeling pretty pumped about all this new stuff in your head and are ready to put it into practice. We'll cover step by step how to focus on what you need and how to do it. Can you skip right to this section? Sure you can, but psychologists tell us that understanding *why* you should do something helps you stick with the plan. Reading about what to do won't help you; doing it will. Remember, you run because you like it and it's fun, right? I want to help you keep on keepin' on.

Let's dive in, shall we? Thanks for reading!

—Jay Dicharry

1

Run Like an Athlete

Running is pure. You may run for yourself, seeking to improve your time on your local neighborhood loop, or maybe simply to knock out the stresses of daily life. Perhaps you run for your country, seeking to set a record in the Olympic coliseum. There are few other sports in the world in which you can compare yourself purely against the clock. It's just you covering distance against time.

And herein lies the catch. It's *you* running against the clock. Or perhaps it's *your athlete* that you coach, or you are helping *your patient* to resume training for their next personal best. Information for runners has been tailored to the advancement of training the heart and lungs—the body's *engine*. You could fill an abyss in the ocean's floor with all the information available to help runners and coaches understand the physiology of running. No matter your personal bias or interpretation of this knowledge base, it plays a significant role in your training your *engine*. However, engines—even big ones—don't move on their own.

Like most kids from the Nintendo generation, I grew up playing my share of games. I liked racing games when I was a kid and a lot of them followed a similar format. They start you off with a simple car for your first race. As you improve your skill on the racetrack, you win races and get "money" that you can use to upgrade your car. It's pretty simple really. Spending your prize money on a bigger engine means you can hit very high speeds. Hey, it's fun to go fast, right? However, you soon realize that all that horsepower leads to a crazy bucking bull in the corners. You just

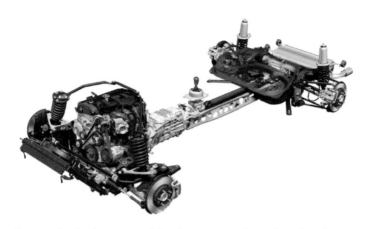

Engines develop horsepower. More horsepower is better, but it's useless unless it is sent to the wheels through a stable chassis.

can't keep it stable in the turns unless you spend some dollars on suspension and tires. The video game almost "forces" you to follow a well-rounded progression of your car because sinking all of your dollars into one category doesn't give you what you need to win the race. It's not just virtual reality—talk to any rally or auto racer and they'll tell you firsthand that they spend more time tuning their suspension and tires than they do on their engine. All of that horsepower needs to be transferred through a *stable chassis* if you want to see the fruits of your labor.

Apparently, most runners didn't play video games back then because running has turned into some crazy type of badge-of-courage sport in which you have to pound yourself into shape day in and day out until you emerge on top. Most runners don't spend time working on their chassis because Coach simply expects more and more miles. There is one incredibly *big* problem with this idea that more is always better. *It's not true.* That's right. How can anyone make this statement?

1. Eighty-two percent of runners get injured. That's an astounding statistic, isn't it? Eighty-two percent of you reading this book will sustain a running–related injury. If eighty-two percent of drivers were getting in wrecks each year, we'd see some pretty major things happen to prevent all these folks from getting hurt, right? So you go see a clinician to get help, and what do you hear? Unless your clinician is a runner himself, like other clinicians, he thinks all runners are nuts. You are told that

"running is bad for you" and you should stop. Since *this has never been proven true*, maybe we should reexamine our approach towards running injuries. Maybe it's time to educate ourselves a bit more on what running really does to the body so you can better prepare—and stay healthy.

2. We're not doing that great on the international scene. We are the biggest, most powerful country in the world . . . yadda yadda yadda . . . yet we don't prove it on the international running scene. Sure, we have our share of standout athletes. The U.S. is really good at putting a million bucks of research and development behind one runner every four years to make sure that we have someone on the Olympic podium to represent us. But that doesn't help *you*, and it doesn't help the millions of other runners in this country. Other nations—nations with a fraction of the global prestige, spending power, and resources—are not just creating occasional standouts, but running *dynasties*. Look at any race distance and the story is always the same. The U.S. will have one or two runners running under a certain time for a certain event. Then look at some of the African nations. They'll have so many runners capable of meeting this time standard, they practically need a waiting list. What is it about the development of runners from overseas that enables them to succeed? Certainly there are some physiological differences, but there are also significant differences in their chassis that we need to explore. Western nations sit and play video games and then run, and then they run more and more. The person running the most number of miles per week does not automatically get a gold medal. *More is not always better.* We have to work from the ground up to build more skilled runners with better control of their body.

Recently, headlines have focused on evolving trends in barefoot running, footwear, and "proprietary" one–for–everyone running form. Thankfully, these headlines have given runners reason to think about running technique. However, somewhere along the line, someone forgot about the individual runner. While moving the runner forward against the clock is what counts, it's *how* the body uses its chassis to stabilize in the lateral and rotational planes to move forward that affects our injury and performance potential. This book is aimed at redirecting that focus. You'll understand how your anatomy works together to answer common questions and become a better runner.

Anatomy for Runners will target your inner *athlete*. While there are many ways to define the term *athlete*, an athlete should be the best they can be at responding to training, accommodating to a variety of external conditions, and performing at their highest level. Let's look beyond running for a second. If you ask the general public, "Who's the greatest athlete of all time?" Michael Jordan's name pops up an awful lot. Why? What is it about Michael Jordan that attracts so much attention? Jordan trained hard to run fast down the court and had the endurance to do this for hours. He had amazing ball-handling skills, an outstanding vertical jump, and the mental calmness to make free throws in noisy arenas. Any single one of these skills is tough to master, but Jordan combined all of them while going up against the best of his peers. A great athlete rises to the occasion and is ready to perform. They not only train their engine, they train the chassis to be able to control their body when running, diving, and jumping.

Most kids are outstanding athletes. Kids learn through play; they learn to run, dive, jump, crawl, climb monkey bars, swing, etc. They explore their limits and refine their movements. They are captains of the playground, developing their motor skills to respond to whatever challenge confronts them. They learn how stiff their legs should be to absorb the motion as they run over the wobbly bridges on the playground, and how much power they must produce to stabilize their body as they jump off the highest step in the front of the house. Their focus is on building muscle memory through play and exploration.

Most runners do not often explore their limits and are not outstanding *athletes*. If you don't agree with this statement, try the following exercise. Grab a video camera or your Smartphone and set it up on a table. Aim it so that you'll be able to walk in front of it and see your full body in frame. Hit record. Walk into view of the camera and do the following test: Put your hands on you hips and stand on your right leg for 30 seconds. Stand on your left leg for 30 seconds. Then go back onto your right leg and close your eyes for 30 more seconds. Finally, 30 seconds on the left leg with eyes closed. If you really want to prove your skill, film yourself jumping up and down on one leg for 30 seconds. Congratulations—you are done with the test. *Stop reading.* Shut the book. Go try this test. It will only take two minutes. Yes, this means you—*stop reading and do the test.* Reading this book is a learning experience only if you apply it.

OK—now that you are done, replay the video. Watch yourself in single-leg balance with eyes open. How stable do you look? Do you shift your trunk around a lot? Do you wobble around on your foot? Compare standing on one leg to standing on the other. Now look at the difference when your eyes were closed. Can you even last 30 seconds without touching your opposite foot down? Are your arms flying around like a Cessna spinning out of control in the air? Do you hop around a lot? Are you able to keep the foot flat on the ground? Do you notice a significant change in your balance when you close your eyes? Why is this harder? When you do the single-leg jumping, can you even do this for 30 seconds continually? Do you hop all over the place or stay generally in one spot?

What does single-leg balance have to do with running? Running is just moving the body's center of mass forward while doing a bunch of single-leg squats. Single-leg balance is pretty close to the single-leg stance phase of running. How did you look during your test? You *did* do the test, didn't you? If balancing was hard enough and balancing while doing the single-leg hop was harder, it's harder yet to balance when running. Why? When running, you are faced with forces of about two and a half times your body weight, plus you fatigue, over time. Still feeling good about your single-leg balance test? Running introduces a lot of repetitive motion in a single plane. These repetitive loads affect the body's tissues. The individual response of tissues in the body will come later, but there is a skill to holding the body stable in the stance phase.

Running is a skill. Kids do lots of dynamic sports that develop varied movement skills. As we move on in life, we begin to narrow our training focus. We do less of the "other stuff" and more running. Then we do even more running. And still, more running. Running is a great way to strengthen the cardiovascular system and the muscles that move us forward in one plane. However, running does not directly strengthen the muscles that stabilize us in the lateral and rotational planes. These muscles are critical with respect to injury and performance potential. We create imbalance as the muscles that propel us forward get a much larger training stimulus to improve than the muscles that stabilize us. The more time and focus we give to one thing, the worse we get at everything else.

Revisiting the aspect of skill, when was the last time you did any running form drills? Look at every other sport and you'll see athletes seeking to refine their movements. Golfers, high jumpers, swimmers, rowers, climbers, tennis players all spend time on improving their sport. What are you doing for your running form? A large number of coaches, clinicians, experts, and runners think that you'll "find" your natural running form with higher mileage. There is evidence to show that higher miles-per-week runners have improved economy as compared to lower mileage runners. However, there are two problems here. First, this assumes that the runner is a perfect athlete. It assumes they have full mobility, full strength, and excellent recruitment of their strength in their running technique. What if this runner is running their weekly volume with a soft tissue mobility restriction that is causing a significant compensation to their gait? They may be running the best they can with their current body, but maybe it's their musculoskeletal system that needs attention. Unless you check for this, it goes unnoticed, untreated, and negatively affects your running. You might improve a given characteristic of your body and need to do drills to incorporate that new ability into your form. In other chapters, we will screen for these mobility and strength limitations and examine the impact of form on running. Secondly, I do not know of any athletes in any other sport that assume they are *that good* to ignore form in their training. Michael Phelps still does drills in the pool during every workout. So does every other athlete at the top of his or her game.

The idea of skill being an important aspect of running may put a lot of folks out of their comfort zone. A lot of the resistance to focusing on form has to do with ignorance of what running form is and how modifications affect it. Laird Hamilton, a professional big-wave surfer, embodies this concept like no other athlete. You see, Laird is routinely faced with waves that are over sixty feet high. The consequences of errors at his stage of the game aren't insignificant, like a sprained ankle. Many surfers at this level attend the funerals of their peers. Laird has arguably the best training philosophy: "Train for what you *don't* know." You may not ever find yourself in a situation where catching the edge of your foot on your board would result in you being pummeled with a fifty-plus foot surf and thrown down to the bottom of the ocean floor. However, I'm willing to bet that each of you has tried to close out your last 400 meters or last mile of a run strongly, only to find that your form fell apart and you couldn't deliver the speed you were after. Maybe this resulted in soreness the day after, or worse yet, an injury. Wouldn't it be nice to know what allowed this to occur, and better yet, what to focus on to prevent this from occurring again?

Finally, while the sexy side of running always leads to talk of personal bests, let's also talk about long-term health. Sure I want you to run fast, but I also want you to have your own knees at age sixty-five. Currently, there is zero evidence that running is harmful to the body. In fact there is work to show that a moderate volume of running is beneficial for joints. However, this assumes that you are running correctly for your body. Prior injuries and the resulting compensations that occur from injuries, mobility deficits, strength losses, and form changes through fatigue all compound your injury risk and produce changes in wear and tear on the body.

The sport of running demands that you bring certain physical attributes and skills to the table. If all you do is run, a lack of one or more of these qualities sends you down the wrong path; unfortunately, most runners don't know where they need to focus their efforts to get back on the right path. This starts right now. You'll learn what types of stresses running places on your body, how the body adapts to stress, and its impact on your biomechanics. You'll apply these concepts with screening tools to identify where you fall short, and more importantly, you'll learn how to fix the weak links in your chain. Runners run, and oftentimes aimlessly, which leads to injury or suboptimal performance. Athletes develop their brain, their body, and the complementary skills necessary to take the right path. Runners, it's time to develop your inner *athlete*.

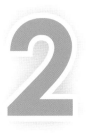

Baby Biomechanics— The Physics of Running

Newton is pissed.
And he's coming after you.

What causes injuries? Most runners don't sustain major traumatic events like falling off of a cliff. The thing that gets runners is compounding *microtraumatic* loads applied to the body mile after mile. Sometimes we ramp up volume too quickly, add too much high intensity work without enough rest, and then we keep pushing through the soreness, aches, and pains, and end up limping. Does this sound familiar? Likely all of you have been guilty! Well, guess what. Your body keeps putting up with your stupidity until it can't anymore. The F.I.T. (Frequency, Intensity, and Time) are just too high to allow proper adaptation of the body's musculoskeletal structure. What does this mean? If we respect the properties of tissue mechanics, we'll better cope with keeping things intact. A training plan that is not set up for individual progression, or one that ignores the mechanical nature of the body's tissues, results in overuse injury.

Sometimes it's not what we do to the body that causes injury (like following a bad training plan), but rather a breakdown within the runner. Perhaps they don't have enough mobility at a specific joint, which forces excessive motion at another joint. Maybe a muscle imbalance prevents them from stabilizing the body. Or it may be a limp that has crept its way into their stride over the years of which they are unaware. Any one of these can act independently or in combination to load the body excessively. It's time to shift our focus to a concept called *causative biomechanics*, and it's the aim of the rest of this book.

Injured runners typically are told to "rest" or follow the typical advice of RICE (Rest, Ice, Compression, and Elevation). While resting/RICE are great strategies for acute injuries or some injuries like fractures, they rarely serve a purpose in long-term management, correcting the reason for the specific injury, or prevention. So many runners "wait around for things to get better and go away." Why not take the bull by the horns? Find out why you got hurt and fix that problem while waiting for the symptoms to subside. We are not talking about cross-training; we'll cover that in a bit. We are talking about correcting the biomechanical factors that caused you to develop your injury in the first place. Even having an injury that requires complete rest is not an excuse. I often have runners working on corrective exercises well before they are back on their feet. If you understand the *specific* factors causing your injury, you can often speed the healing rate and often emerge a better athlete than you were prior to the injury. If this sounds like a good idea to you, let's dive in together.

It's understood that a specific F.I.T. of training is required to improve the cardiovascular system—the engine. Athletes tailor their training to improve specific outcomes, or limiters. If you want to improve your endurance, the priority shifts to longer distance training at lower intensities so that the body can improve its ability to transport oxygen and utilize fat as an energy substrate. Likewise, if top-end speed is the goal, the emphasis shifts towards higher intensity work with long rest between repetitions so that intensity can be maintained for the duration of the workout. Training is targeted towards specific *central* and *peripheral* adaptations. *Central adaptations* refer to the ability to carry more oxygen and nutrients to working tissue. *Peripheral adaptations* occur inside the local muscles to improve the extraction and utilization of the oxygen and energy substrates delivered. Just as there is a science that governs the principles that we use to develop the engine, there is a science that governs the development of the chassis.

To optimize the training adaptations of the chassis, the stresses on the tissues need to be kept within their optimal window. Training loads create a stimulus for the body to help you heal and emerge a stronger you. Wolf's Law states that tissues in the body adapt to the loads placed upon them. Training breaks the body down. If the rate of recovery matches the rate of breakdown,

Effect of Physical Stress on Tissue Adaptation

Physical stress level →	Death
	Injury
	Increased tolerance (hypertrophy)
	Maintenance
	Decreased tolerance (atrophy)
	Death

the body will maintain its current state. To improve the connective tissues that make up the chassis, the load needs to be increased to some point. When the training load falls on either side of the optimal, the repair process is compromised. If the load is too high, such that the body cannot fully recover prior to the next workout, breakdown can occur. Likewise, too little activity can result in the body's tissues becoming weaker. This is why simply resting doesn't always yield stronger tissues. Further, not every tissue in the body adapts at the same rate. Sometimes the body needs to be assisted to help it repair correctly. Specific loading of tissues helps the body repair.

An all-too-common scenario: Paul is a high school runner living in the city who has been carefully ramping up his training volume over the summer to develop a solid base for the fall cross-country season. His workouts have stressed his body appropriately so that he is able to remodel his body at a steady level for the resultant breakdown that occurs with training. This concept has kept him within the "optimal window." Four weeks prior to the start of fall classes, Paul heads to the scenic mountains to attend a running camp. Here, Paul is challenged with vastly different terrain than his body is used to. Further, his teammates and athletes from other schools are running slightly quicker than Paul is used to. The combination of challenging terrain and slightly faster paces during workouts fatigues Paul to the point where he compensates his gait pattern. The mechanical stresses acting on his body are different from those he had all summer and push him outside of the optimal window. Paul is breaking his body down faster than he can recover. By the time camp is over, he has developed pain in his Achilles. Paul returns home and informs his coach that he has pain that is almost too severe to allow him to run. The coach advises Paul to stop running to rest the ankle. Paul respects the advice of his coach and stops running. He also stops all other athletic activity and is determined to be 100 percent by the start of the season—just three weeks away.

Paul's inactivity over the next few weeks helps the pain subside. He begins to lose focus and gets busy with his summer job and girlfriend. He figures that all the training he did at the beginning of the season is enough to prepare him. While rest can allow inflammation to reduce, he does nothing at all over this period of inactivity. His body is now receiving an insufficient stimulus and actually begins to decondition. The mechanical structures that make up his body actually begin to weaken, even though Paul is now symptom-free.

School is back in session and Paul joins his teammates for workouts. Since the majority of the team had been consistently training all summer long and had a successful training camp, they arrive in better shape than Paul. Paul jumps right back in and pushes things a bit too quickly. Within two weeks, the Achilles symptoms have resumed, and he is now forced to miss the first four races of the season. He sees the school's trainer and receives ice and electric stimulation to help reduce the swelling and his symptoms, but he's not improving.

Does this situation sound familiar to you? If not, replace the words "high school" with "college." Or replace the "early high school season" with your transition to 5K and 10K training after marathon season. Replace "summer job"

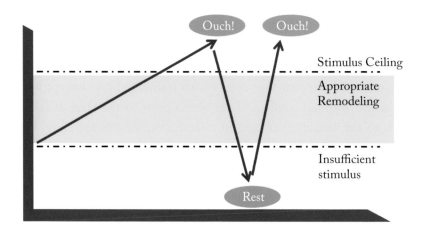

Optimal running adaptations occur when the training stimulus is in the appropriate window. Paul bounces around with too high and too low of a consistent stimulus, leading to poor outcomes.

with "career," and swap "girlfriend" for "wife/husband." Given that 82 percent of runners are injured, the chances that you or your runner could have auditioned for Paul's role in this story are exceptionally high. If you were cast as Paul, what would you have done differently? Would you have rested completely? Maintained a reduced running volume? Would you have changed shoes? Would you have iced the leg more or less? Would you have done any corrective stretches or exercises while waiting for the area to heal? Cross-training? Are the answers to any of the above questions informed or based on the lore passed down through your friends? Before you can correctly answer any of these questions, it's essential to understand *microanatomy* and how the tissues of the body respond to different *mechanical stresses*.

Mechanical Properties

The body is primarily made up of something called *collagen*. It's configured differently in the body for different purposes. Just as trees have different parts that developed from the same seed, you have different parts that developed from . . . well . . . that's another book entirely! Collagen is very strong stuff. It approaches the tensile strength of steel, yet it's highly flexible. The structural organization of the collagen fibers produces different properties. Depending on

Tissue Specificity

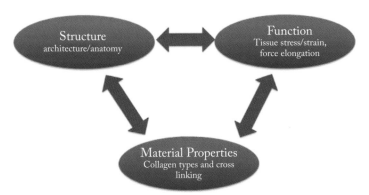

Form determines function, but the tissues also develop and optimize based on their use. For example, the fibers in a muscle may have a given structural architecture, but the repetitive stresses they see during running may cause adaptations that shorten and excessively bind layers of tissues together that impact their overall function. To restore this, you must fix the tissue properties, but also address the mechanical cause that altered the tissue in the first place.

An electron micrograph of healthy collagen fibers. When multiple collagen strands, or a group of straws, run together, they function as one and the net strength is much stronger.

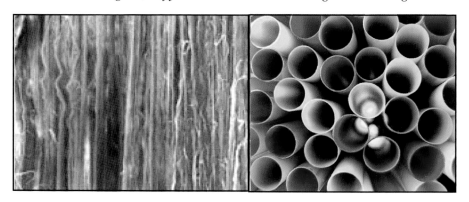

the tissue, this orientation can be specialized to provide resistance to force, tension, stretch, compression, pressure, elasticity, or any combination thereof.

All collagen fibers within a single tissue are specifically aligned so that they can respond to specific loads. The electron micrograph above shows healthy collagen fibers running parallel to each other in the same linear direction. This arrangement is similar to straws in a box. Each individual straw is a cylinder that can support load in one direction very well, at the expense of supporting load from another direction. If you hold a straw upright on the table, you can push pretty hard before it buckles. However, if you pinch the sides together, it takes almost no force to collapse the straw. You want the straw oriented so that it can best respond to the kind of stress it will see, and bundling several straws together produces a very strong tissue. You could likely place a five- or ten-pound weight directly on top of the straws in the box without any straws buckling under the load. The orientation of collagen fibers makes it possible for your connective tissues to deal with incredibly high forces that they will deal with in sports like running.

Various mechanical factors impact the collagen formation in the body during running. Working definitions of these specific factors will provide a solid foundation to explore the mechanical changes that occur in the body. Following the definition, we'll apply these terms to an example.

- **Stress:** The force per cross-sectional area of a given object.
- **Strain:** The amount of deformation that occurs (defined in the percent change in length).

Stress Strain

With stress, a force is applied to a tissue, but there is no change in length. Strain means that the force was high enough to physically alter the position of the tissue.

Types of Stress and Strain

- **Compression:** Forces are applied in the same line and in the same direction.
- **Tension:** Forces applied in the same line, but opposite direction.
- **Shear:** Force applied in parallel lines, but opposite direction.

Two objects are on a table. On the left is a brick. On the right is a "brick" of silly putty with the same length, width, and height as the real brick. Imagine now that we place a ten-pound weight on top of the brick. Nothing really happens to the brick. The ten-pound weight is applying a given amount of *stress* to the brick. Since stress refers to the force per area applied, the size of the brick would increase or decrease the size of the stress being applied to the brick. Nonetheless, the material composition of the brick is oriented to withstand *compression*. The brick does not bend or lengthen and is not under significant *strain* (change in length). Let's now apply the exact same ten–pound weight to the silly putty brick. When applying the exact same stress (the ten–pound weight) to the exact same cross-sectional area (same size), the silly putty undergoes a lot of deformation. It changes its configuration based on the *stress* applied and undergoes significant *strain*.

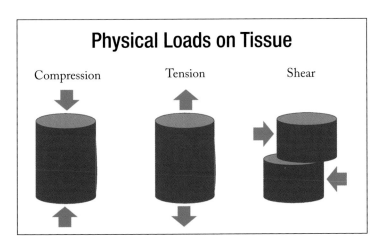

Physical Loads on Tissue

Compression   Tension   Shear

Based on these results, one might presume that the real brick is stronger than the silly putty brick. One must be careful when drawing this conclusion. Let's look at another example. Imagine a *tensile* load trying to pull the brick apart. While bricks are very strong under *compression*, it doesn't take nearly as much force to break them in half as pulling them apart. And when the brick breaks, it's into several pieces—completely destroyed. This is similar to a fracture in a bone. The exact same *tensile* stress applied to the silly putty brick would lengthen the silly putty, but not result in a catastrophic failure and fractured pieces. This is similar to what might occur in a muscle belly. Thus we can conclude that the real brick holds better under compressive loads, and the silly putty holds better under tensile loads. The same principle holds true in your body. Tissues are specialized in the way that they respond to external and internal stress during running.

The Load-Deformation Curve

Just as the architecture of the respective tissue affects the way it responds to running, different amounts of force result in different internal changes in the tissues. The graph below plots the increase in load against deformation of the tissue.

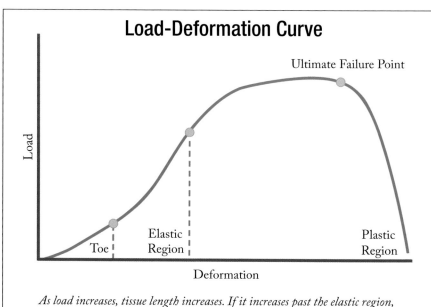

Load-Deformation Curve

Ultimate Failure Point

Load

Toe | Elastic Region | Plastic Region

Deformation

As load increases, tissue length increases. If it increases past the elastic region, the tissue is changed. This could be negative (chronic overload can break down tissues) or positive (stretching into this range to increase length).

- **Load:** force applied to a structure. Tissue response is dependent on magnitude, direction, and rate of application.
- **Deformation:** change in configuration of the tissue when force applied.
- **Toe:** the change in length of the tissue where slack is taken up.
- **Elastic Region:** the deformation will not be permanent when the load is removed (reversible).
- **Plastic Region:** deformation will be permanent when the load is removed; this leads to microfailure.
- **Ultimate Failure Point:** the load was so overwhelming that it resulted in microfailure.

Let's see how all the technical stuff above comes together in the real world during a hamstring stretch. Imagine lying on the floor with your knees bent to ninety degrees and your feet flat on the floor. At rest, the collagen fibers that make up the muscle and tendon are not 100 percent straight. Under no load and in a shortened position, they are slightly crimped, similar to a herringbone pattern. With your knees bent, feel your hamstrings—they'll feel loose and are very pliable. Now begin to straighten one knee out so that the leg lies flat on the floor. While you won't feel any stretch, you've lengthened the muscles just enough to take up the slack in the hamstrings. This is what occurs during the "toe" period. Nothing really occurs other than the taking up of slack, or smoothing out the wrinkles. Now, keeping the knee straight, flex the hip to lift the leg up towards the ceiling. As your leg gets further off of the ground, you'll notice the onset of a slight stretch in the hamstrings. The fibers in the muscle are tensing as you increase the length. Hold your leg in this position for about 10–15 seconds and then return it to the ground. What you've just done is take the hamstring muscles through the elastic range. You applied a force sufficient to lengthen them temporarily. But, when the leg was brought back down, the force was removed, and the hamstrings returned to their original length. The hamstrings did not receive enough of a stimulus to permanently change their length.

Let's repeat this experiment. Raise the leg up again to the point where you feel the onset of stretch (the elastic region) and continue to the point at which you feel a moderate stretch. Hold this position for three full minutes, and then return the leg to the ground. The combination of a greater load (more length plus more time) pushed the hamstrings into the plastic region.

The muscle received enough load to result in microtears in the muscle belly, which resulted in a physical change in length. The hamstring muscles are now longer than they were prior to the stretch. If the goal was in fact to lengthen the hamstring due to tightness, then a beneficial change has resulted. Later in this book we'll dig deeper into stretching and why this may or may not be a good thing. OK, last part of the experiment. Don't actually do this one, though! Imagine that you repeated the above exercise, taking the leg back into the plastic range, and then pushed even deeper into a stretch. Just at this moment, your friend runs over to you and throws his entire body weight onto your overly lengthened hamstring. There is an excellent chance that the combination of terminal length and a high force will take your hamstring to the ultimate failure point and result in a significant tear of the muscle belly. Again, don't try this at home!

The above criteria apply to more than stretching. Loads are a combination of change in length and forces that affect the musculoskeletal system. The take-home message is that loads into and out of the elastic region don't really change any of the physical properties of the tissue and thus don't generate a large stimulus to the body to make a change. Loads that take us into the plastic region will result in a permanent change in the tissue, and spark some type of repair process to bring the tissue back to a new "baseline." Loads that take us to the ultimate failure point result in significant damage to the structure. In some cases this damage requires rest with immobilization to allow the body to repair, and in other cases may require casting or surgery. Training loads that fluctuate in the elastic region and occasionally mildly in the plastic region are appropriate stresses to bring about positive changes in the runner. Loads that move well into the plastic region typically result in acute or chronic problems that should not be part of a smart training plan.

Stiffness is defined as load (stress) divided by deformation (strain). Put more simply, it's how resistant a tissue is to changing its length when a load is applied to it. Stiffness is not a negative tissue trait; it's an inherent property of the body that we must be aware of when examining how training affects the runner.

Numerous factors affect a tissue's adaptation to stiffness:

- Disuse results in smaller and fewer collagen fibers, resulting in decreased strength and stiffness. These changes negatively affect the body's ability to deal with running. This is why you feel "weak" after taking a long break from running—you are!

- Increased use promotes remodeling to improve strength and stiffness, as long as modifications to F.I.T. are progressive. In chronically over-loaded injuries, an increase in F.I.T. is associated with a decrease in the ultimate strength of the tissue and will impair healing. While rest or relative rest may be important to let inflammation subside, a moder-ated F.I.T. of loading during rehab is critical to prepare for a full return to participation. The F.I.T. during rehab should be enough to promote healing, but not enough to impair it. If you are confused, seek out pro-fessional help. Physical therapists do this type of work for a living; you likely don't.

- Tissues that have more elastic fibers can tolerate more load without moving into the plastic region. Their load-deformation plots have a flatter curve and are less stiff.

- A proper warm-up improves blood flow and elevates the tissue temper-ature of working muscles. This makes it easier to accommodate stress and strain during the run. Therefore, a physiologic warm-up at low intensity has merit prior to full efforts.

- The natural aging process yields a decreased ability to adapt to high stress. This is due to reduced vascularity (blood supply) and reduced number and activity of reparative cells. An older runner's tissues become stiffer and less able to tolerate a given workload. Assuming identical F.I.T. for an older and younger runner, the stiffer musculoskeletal struc-ture of the older runner will be stressed more than the younger runner's.

- The rate at which tissues are loaded affects stiffness. Some tissues, such as cartilage, are more affected by how quickly they are loaded than oth-ers. In general though, all the tissues in the body are *viscoelastic*: more resistant to change the faster the rate is applied. This increase in stiff-ness allows the tissues to remain intact under the high forces and short stance times during your run.

The inflammatory cycle plays a major role in initiating the healing process. Traditionally, swelling has been viewed as a negative event with a significant number of runners popping anti-inflammatories as often as vitamins. However, swelling is very important at both the microscopic (cellular) and macroscopic levels. When faced with damage, the cells signal a host of chemicals that act as messengers. These messengers spread the word that something is in fact wrong, and an entire cascade of events is set in motion to repair the damaged tissue. At the macroscopic level, swelling is the body's natural attempt to "splint" the body part. The increased extracellular fluid that is drawn in as the result of swelling acts to increase pressure around the area to minimize stress to the affected tissue. Swelling increases our pain sensitivity around the area, which is helpful since you will strive to lessen the load on the affected tissue. The body's natural responses are not so dumb; listening to them will result in proper healing.

Unfortunately, traditional medicine has not *listened* to the body, but tried to *silence* it. The cellular messengers that were mentioned above are critical to begin the inflammatory process. If we cover their mouths, they can't spread the word. Taking non-steroidal anti-inflammatories, such as Ibuprofen and Naproxen, suppresses the messenger chemicals from "calling in the troops." Instead of calling in the army, only a few friends show up to help. Further, these over-the-counter medications block the pain receptors, meaning you ignore the fact that the area is dysfunctional and continue to load it. This excessive stress prevents the tissue from healing. If your pesky older brother hits you in the same spot on your arm each and every day, the ongoing tissue damage prevents you from

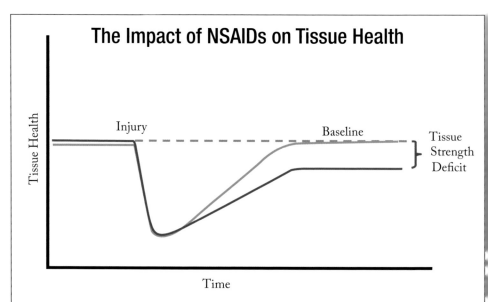

The body will always try to heal. Chronic usage of NSAIDs impacts the repair process and prevents healing back to baseline tissue strength. This weaker, impaired tissue is now at a greater risk for reinjury.

healing. Just as feeling the constant pain would lead you to run away from your brother to stop the ongoing tissue stress, feeling the pain in the injured body part would encourage you to minimize stress to the injured area. The swelling and pain suppression from NSAIDs (non-steroidal anti-inflammatory drugs) results in a delayed and slower healing response than would have been possible without the NSAIDs.

Of course the formal disclaimer is that you should first and foremost check with your doctor about the need for medications; however, it is safe to say that the tide is changing. We live in a society of "now." You take a pill so that you can continue training today. Most sports medicine specialists are no longer recommending NSAIDs for acute injuries. Newer research has shown that while you may squeak in a bit of extra training time taking NSAIDs, the healing will take longer and will not be as complete as if you left the cap on the pill bottle. This substandard state is less able to cope with training loads. Further, there is strong evidence to show that NSAIDs may significantly delay the healing of bone.

So, no NSAIDs . . . what about ice? NSAIDs try to suppress the initiation of the inflammatory cycle from ever beginning. Ice acts differently and has no effect on the messenger activation process. Icing the area serves to minimize the swelling that is there. Ice speeds the removal of the extracellular fluid around the injured area and thus helps clear the waste products of the repair process away from the injury site.

Let's apply these principles using a hamstring strain. By definition, a muscle strain is a partial or complete tear of the muscle belly. The hamstring receives abnormal tensile loads resulting in a change in strain distribution in the muscle and/or tendon. The normal collagen alignment is disrupted, and the messenger chemicals in the blood signal new materials to report for duty and rebuild the damage site. The initiation of the inflammatory process gets the body's healing response rolling. However, this healing rate is compounded by certain things that we may or may not do. Let's take a look:

- **F.I.T.**–Is the dosage of training enough to allow the body to heal? Perhaps the runner can continue to train through this injury, running 50 percent of their previous volume. Perhaps they can continue to train at full volume, only limiting the speed. Or maybe complete rest is required. These training adjustments must be selected on an individual basis, but some adaptation must be made to allow proper healing.

Continuing to train full volume and full speed on an injured area will result in tissue breaking down faster than its capacity to heal. A lot of runners walk the tightrope—they never fully recover from their initial injury and continue to overload the body just to the point where they are teetering on reinjury. F.I.T. should be modified to allow healing.

- **Cross-training**–The best way to train for running is to train by running. However, the weight-bearing aspect of running increases the mechanical forces of the body to the point where the tissue can't heal. Using limited or reduced weight-bearing activities can allow the runner to continue to train the engine while reducing the mechanical tissue stress on the injury site. Common forms are elliptical, cycling, walking, water-running, and reduced gravity environment treadmills. The research on cross-training shows that the *central adaptations* that occur in the body are maintained and can even be improved with cross-training. It's the *peripheral adaptations* that are best served by actually running. Again, keep the F.I.T. in mind when designing the cross-training activity and volume. Try to pick an activity you are more familiar with. If your prior run volume was 30 miles per week, now is not the time to start cycling 180 miles per week. As crazy as it sounds, this occurs frequently with motivated runners. All activities place some stress on the body. The correct formula for cross-training is enough volume to maintain the central adaptations while minimizing the stress to the injured area. After all, the goal is to heal and resume running!

- **Nutrition**–Americans send more vitamins down the toilet than their bodies can absorb. If you eat a reasonably balanced diet and live in the modern Western world, you likely get enough vitamins and minerals. There is no rationale for every injured athlete to take any specific supplement. However, signs that you are not healing at the expected rate are a red flag. Contact your physician for further evaluation to see if you do have any specific needs that are not being met by your current diet.

- **Sleep**–Exactly how much sleep you need varies on an individual basis. However, most research recommends seven to nine hours of sleep for optimal function. Not just optimal function of your brain, but also optimal repair and regeneration of your body.

Let's assume that the runner with the hamstring strain cut back his volume, is getting lots of sleep and a good diet, and is on his way to eliminating his symptoms. In another chapter, we'll cover the exact mechanics that cause hamstring strain, but let's review the repair process of the torn muscle and tendon. The body repairs the tissue with scar formation. Through the rehab process, all he did was continue running at a reduced volume and stretched for one minute daily. After being pain-free for three weeks, he is cleared to resume to full speed and work his way back to full volume. Things appear to be going well for a few weeks.

After three weeks of running at full intensity, his symptoms return. This time, he decides to give the injury a proper evaluation. Upon assessing his hamstring muscle belly, areas of significant fibrosis (trigger points) are found throughout his lateral hamstrings. The tear did repair itself after the initial injury; however, it repaired in a very disorganized fashion. All of his collagen fibers, or "straws," aren't oriented in the same direction, making the repair less able to withstand the stresses in running. The "healed" tissue is significantly weaker than it was preinjury, making reinjury likely. Unless the tissue mechanics are restored, this poor state of healing will persist. Two key interventions can be employed to improve the organization of the tissue:

1. Free up the straws. When the collagen fibers don't point in the same direction, they point all over at random. These nonlinear bonds become stiff and limit mobility. In Chapter 5, we'll cover this in depth. For now, we'll simply state that the goal is to break up the sticky stuff that is binding down the body.
2. Give them a reason to align back into parallel formation by doing eccentric exercises. Wolf's Law states that the body improves when faced with tensile forces in the line of stress of the tissue. Step one is to break up the scar fibers that don't lie in the same direction; the aim of step two is to get the scar fibers to lay down in the direction they should. *Eccentric* means "lengthening under active contraction," which is similar to a "negative" if you've ever spent time in the weight room. If not, try this. Lift up a gallon of milk. Then very, very slowly lower it. Even though the muscles are getting longer, they are actively working to slow the milk jug down against gravity. Eccentric activity orients stress through the muscle and tendon and encourages the body to lay

down collagen fibers to better produce and accommodate forces inside the connective tissue architecture. In the case of a hamstring strain, this is accomplished by doing double- and single-leg dead lifts or eccentric hip extension with progressive increases in volume and resistance.

The goal of healing any injury is always optimal repair. The running-specific goal is to get the athlete training back at full volume. In this example case, running at a reduced volume, gentle stretching, and time were sufficient enough to allow some repair of the muscle strain. However, those same adjustments did not encourage *ideal* recovery of the tissue properties, resulting in rapid reinjury. Rest, or relative rest, doesn't always yield stronger tissues. Sometimes the body needs to be assisted to help it repair correctly. Specific loading of the tissue along the lines of stress maximizes the repair process. If the focus was optimizing the tissue function from the onset, the chances of reinjury could have been significantly reduced. Research has even shown that preventative eccentric training can reduce the chance of sustaining a muscle strain. Instead of focusing solely on the return to running, the aim should be to determine what unique mechanical factors caused the injury and normalize the tissue repair along the timeline. This makes the difference between missing your race and running it successfully.

Can I run through an injury?

The goal is always the same: to ensure that the body is able to build up faster than training is breaking it down. Dr. Bob Wilder's *Rules for Runners* makes simple use of the information covered above:

1. On a 10-point scale, pain during the run should be no greater than 0–3.
2. Pain should not be severe to the point where you limp during or following the run.
3. The long run should not be more than half the regular weekly volume.

Summary

While you run about with the wind in your ears, your body is faced with mechanical stresses. If these mechanical stresses overload the tissue, you become injured. While this chapter was technical in nature, a foundation in biomechanics helps you make sense of random advice you'll hear about running. When someone tells you to change something, think about what type of effect that specific change will have on your body. What delays healing? Excessive running, cross-training, impaired endocrine function, and poor nutrition. While the correct amount of rest (reduction in F.I.T.) can decrease stress on the tissue to allow healing, the critical thing here is correct amount. Some tissues just need inactivity. Some need a reduced training load. Some tissues need to be completely unloaded to heal. Poor biomechanics alter the path of stress and strain through the tissues and break things down. The next step in the education process is to take a look at how each of these forces affects the anatomical structures of the musculoskeletal system.

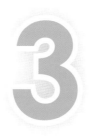

Microanatomy—
What Are You Made Of?

Momma told you that you were special.
Your body's parts are special too.
Let's give them some respect.

Does anyone actually read instructions anymore? You know—that little pamphlet that comes with stuff you buy? How about product specs? Don't check out those either, huh? While our body doesn't come with an instruction book, it does have "specifications" in which the varied tissues respond to the mechanical forces during running. Think of your body from an engineering standpoint. We have all seen signs over bridges with weight limits. The engineers who designed the bridge only rate the particular structure for a certain weight limit due to the strength of the materials involved. If the bridge becomes overloaded, it can't repair itself back to its original state. While body parts don't have signs on them with peak load limits, they have a peak ceiling of load they can tolerate prior to breakdown. Unlike the bridge, your body's parts can heal, and do so at different rates depending on the attributes of the tissue type. Understanding the unique constraints of each tissue type can help promote positive healing. The question should not be: Should I take a week off for my ____ injury? The correct question is: How can I promote positive healing in the impaired tissue? To get the answer, you have to delve into the microanatomy.

There are many types of connective tissues, each having their own architecture or orientation. It's this specific orientation that makes bone respond differently to running than the tendon does. Mechanical forces that speed recovery for some tissues may not be good for others.

Your car's chassis is made up of all kinds of different parts that all have different jobs. Some parts are designed to keep the frame square, some are mobile so that the wheels can turn, and some of them, like springs, absorb forces. Although they are all made of some type of metal, they all have a different job to do.

Your body's chassis has different parts that all serve different functions as well. Although all of the parts are made up of collagen, their fiber alignment, nutrition delivery system, and adaptive capacity set them up to do very different jobs. Functioning together, these different tissues enable movement against the forces of gravity while running, jumping, climbing, and anything else you do. However, the way they tolerate stress, repair themselves, and enable performance at a maximal level is unique to each tissue. The take-home here is that running a certain volume per week doesn't stress everything in the same way. Cross-training doesn't stress everything in the same way. Rest doesn't improve everything at the same rate either. Let's look a bit deeper.

Bone

The bones of the skeleton provide structure. There are 206 bones in the body that serve as the pulleys and levers through which we transmit forces. While they are strong, they do have elasticity and even exhibit a slight flex under load.

There are two general parts to the bone:

1. **Cortical:** This is the outside layer, very similar to the tough candy shell on the outside of M&M's. This dense, compact layer comprises 80 percent of the skeleton and provides support to the internal bone and bone marrow. The attachment points of all the body's tendons and ligaments insert onto this layer.

2. **Cancellous:** Most of us don't eat M&M's purely for the candy coating: we want the good stuff—the chocolate center. Even though the cancellous region of the bone makes up less than 20 percent of the overall

Layers of Bone

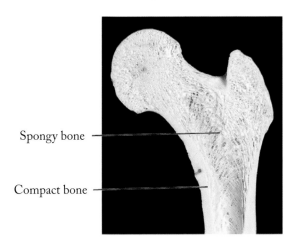

Spongy bone

Compact bone

In this section of the femur, you can easily see the difference between the hard outer layer of bone and the softer, less dense, spongy inner layer.

bone mass, this is where the majority of the activity in the bone occurs. This region is highly metabolically active (lots of tissue turnover) and highly vascular (good blood supply). Take a look at a dry sponge and you'll see that its fibers provide some type of structure, but there is a lot of space between the fibers as well. The inner layer of bone is similar such that the scaffolding of trabeculae fibers is oriented to withstand loads based on the individual bone's alignment and orientation.

About two-thirds of the blood supply to bone comes from dedicated arteries that enter the bone. The remaining one-third of the blood supply comes from offshoots of muscles close to the bone. Internally, blood is distributed within the bone via a highly organized network of vessels, the *Haversian* and *Volkmann's canals.*

Not only does bone provide passive structure and support, it provides an active center for blood cell production and mineral storage. The bone marrow is the center of blood cell production for the entire body. Red blood cells are critical for oxygen transport throughout the body. Storage of calcium inside the bone is constantly regulated and adjusted based on the body's need for calcium's other functions. While calcium is a significant building block for bone, its presence is required for muscle contraction, swelling control, and a host of other cellular functions.

Specific levels of freely circulating and stored calcium are tightly monitored by cells called *osteocytes*. These cells monitor changes in ion exchange (yes—tiny electrical currents), bone turnover, and *mechanosensitivity* to regulate the storage and release of calcium. Bone is constantly in a state of turnover, being broken down and rebuilt. *Osteoblasts* are cells that lay down new bone to increase structural integrity. *Osteoclasts* are cells that break bone down to release calcium into the body for other cellular functions. At any point in time, the dominance of the osteoblast or osteoclast yields either a net buildup or a net breakdown of bone density. The dominance of buildup versus breakdown is governed by the stress load on the bone and the endocrine system (which maintains hormone levels).

Bone is a highly adaptive material that can alter its properties and configuration in response to mechanical demands. Wolf's Law of bone remodeling states: Where there is optimal stress (loading) within bone, deposits of bone occur at a greater rate than bone resorption. Thus the bone becomes stronger. When there is nonoptimal stress (whether from excessive training stress or severe lack of activity, as during bed rest), deposits of bone occur at a lower rate than bone resorption. The bone becomes weaker. Bones respond well to

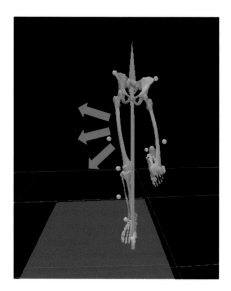

Bones move. While your bones are strong, they are not rigid; they bend, bow, and twist from the forces exerted on them. This example shows a slight lateral bow of the femur during stance, resulting from the ground's reaction force on the inside of the leg.

compressive forces. Controlled, progressive increases in the load applied to the bone through training result in positive adaptations. Bone is the only connective tissue in the body that is capable of repair to 100 percent of its original preinjured state.

The endocrine system controls the hormone levels in the body. The body likes to keep things within a fairly narrow operating range. Hormone levels in the body at any point in time are a response to maintaining controlled levels of activity called *homeostasis* (keeping things status quo). Lying in bed, it's very easy to maintain everything since there is not a significant stress to the body. Training throws a major shift into this well-maintained state. Long runs, speed work, weight sessions, plyometrics, and food intake prior to and after workouts all introduce different levels of variability into this equation and make your body work harder to keep the repair process in check. The endocrine system has an especially large effect on bone health for women.

The Female Athlete Triad syndrome has been the downfall of many a runner. Most women can acknowledge it but are so focused on their next workout or race that they ignore the signs. This diagnosis is highly correlated with both previous and future stress fractures. There are three factors that lead to a downward spiral in the body's ability to recover from the injury:

1. **High exercise volume**—The F.I.T. are too great for the athlete to recover even under ideal conditions.
2. **Poor nutrition**—There are not enough substrates to heal properly from the injury. Body image problems are rampant in runners. If you aren't taking in a minimum amount of calories to maintain proper body weight, you won't just lose fat, you'll lose bone and muscle as well . . . not ideal!
3. **Ammenorhea**—Abnormality in menstrual cycles is a sign that the endocrine system can't keep up. This is both a cause and an effect. The endocrine system is so stressed trying to keep hormones in check that menstrual cycles become irregular. Since the hormone levels are in flux, the signal to repair the body is significantly reduced. Normal menstrual cycles are important to help maintain bone health.

How does this diagnosis typically play out? The Female Athlete Triad is mostly seen in adolescent runners. What two things does this population have in common? A high consumption of dark sodas and poor body image. These sodas have high amounts of phosphates that leech calcium out of the bones. There is no need to soft step around Female Athlete Triad. It's easy to tell a group of teenage girls that sodas are bad for them and convince them to shift their drinking preferences, but it's a bit tougher to tell this same group of girls that they are not overweight. Poor body image is the root of the problem. Eating disorders don't only lead to poor run times, they compromise normal development. Young women are constantly inundated with ads of overly skinny and computer-manipulated virtual models. Carrying around less weight to boost running efficiency compounds this desire to be overly thin. However, skinny does not always equal healthy.

Triad is a major health problem—how are you going to deal with it? Have a plan in place. Yes, many of you have heard this before, but do you actually have the number of a counselor or psychologist in your contact list that you can refer to today? Conquering eating disorders goes well beyond a lecture about the food pyramid—you have to take the entire psychosocial side of body image head on. Reducing volume will de-stress the injured site, but if the nutrition and endocrine aspects are not addressed through behavior modification, the runner will not heal and will likely have far-reaching health effects. Find an expert in your community and don't be afraid to reach out to them.

What if you or your athlete is not healing from the stress fracture? Stress fractures occur from time to time as a result of training errors. People make mistakes; everyone is "allowed" one. After you've been diagnosed with a second stress fracture, it's critical to determine if the issue is more medically related. Your doctor will assess your bone density and endocrine function through various imaging procedures (typically an MRI or a bone scan) and blood tests. The World Health Organization identifies *normal* bone density using T-scores. Normal bone mass is > -1, osteopenia (low bone density) is -1 to -2.5, and osteoporosis is < -2.5. Here's some homework: review your diet. Actually write down what you eat in a given day on a sheet of paper and then look up the calcium contents online. Men should get 1,000 milligrams daily. Women should take in at least 1300 milligrams of calcium daily. If you are deficient, make a focused attempt to alter your intake. Bone healing is also dependent on Vitamin D and iron levels, as well as a host of other things. If you aren't healing, there is likely a reason. Get some help from your physician and figure it out. You have 206 bones to take care of, and it's up to you to ensure they are strong and healthy.

Tendons

Tendons are highly elastic structures that are able to withstand high amounts of tensile forces. The tremendous amount of force that muscles generate is transferred to the bone via the tendon. Tendons play a major role in running by storing and releasing elastic energy to propel the body forward. We'll cover this much deeper in Chapter 8.

Tendons have very little direct blood supply and get most of their nutrition through a sheath that surrounds the tendon containing *synovial fluid*. Repair is due to specialized cells called *fibroblasts* that improve structure and density of the tendon. Through gradual increases in mileage and intensity, the body progressively adapts and disperses stress uniformly throughout the connective tissue structure of the tendon. When a tendon becomes overloaded, it is the result of one or more of the following four major mechanisms which alter the distribution of forces inside the tendon:

1. **Tensile stresses**—Gradual increases in F.I.T. result in a tensile direction of beneficial adaptations. When these tensile loads become too high (either from a sudden change in F.I.T.) or significantly different (from surface or shoe changes that the runner has not adapted to), the tendon can become overwhelmed and weaken.

2. **Friction pulley issues**—There is some amount of friction between any two surfaces. The friction between the tendon and any bony landmarks that it courses around can cause excessive shear force applied to the tendon sheath.

3. **Compression pulley issues**—As the tendon courses around the bony landmark, there is some amount of force acting perpendicular to the tendon that can result in increased compression force to the tendon, and thus impair its ability to move and distribute load throughout its structure. Thus, high strain can result in focal areas of the tendon.

4. **Interface of the musculotendinous junction**—Take a look at Velcro and notice the "hooks" on one side and the "loops" on the other. When pressed together, they form a tight bind. This is similar to the bind between muscle and tendon—there is an interlacing of the fibers. However, it's the respective properties of the tissues that create the issue. Muscles tolerate high-volume, low-load activity well, while tendons prefer low-volume, high-load activity.

Where these two tissue types meet is an area that is compromised in its ability to equally distribute strain.

Tendonitis versus Tendinosis

Tendonitis is a very common, but misleading term, thrown around a lot. If you seek treatment for pain in the tendon and your care provider suggests a corticosteroid injection, run far away! Why? Corticosteroids are drugs that reduce inflammation. They are typically injected along with a small amount of a numbing drug called lidocaine. By definition, anything that ends in "-itis" means "inflammation of." The tendon is inflamed, so let's inject it and calm it down. Sounds great, right? The problem here is that it's not true. *Tendons are not capable of inflammation.* There is no inflammation for the corticosteroid to suppress. In fact, they do bad things to the tendon. Research shows that tendons are *weaker* following corticosteroid injection. To make matters worse, the lidocaine numbs the site and makes the pain go away, so you resume training too quickly. The weakened tissue is subjected to full load before it is ready and you wind up right back to where you started.

Since there is no inflammation in the tendons, there is no such thing as *tendonitis.* There is a term called *tendinosis* that better describes the damage of tendons. By definiton, tendinosis is *chronic degeneration of tendon tissue with reduced collagen fiber content and increased volume of mucoid ground substance with disrupted collagen orientation and an absence of inflammatory cells.* Kind of wordy, right? Basically, look back at the straws example we used in Chapter 2.

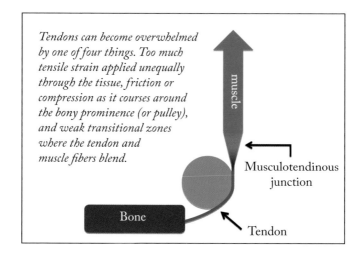

Tendons can become overwhelmed by one of four things. Too much tensile strain applied unequally through the tissue, friction or compression as it courses around the bony prominence (or pulley), and weak transitional zones where the tendon and muscle fibers blend.

muscle

Musculotendinous junction

Bone

Tendon

The random orientation of scar tissue creates stiff spots throughout the tissue. These stiff spots are subject to high levels of strain and become damaged. The long-term fix for tendinosis is to spread out the load inside the tendon so that it is more uniform throughout. Thus, treatment of tendon issues should follow this model:

- **Relative rest**—Decrease tissue load to allow the tendon to heal. This can vary from reduction of volume to cross-training to complete rest based on the extent of injury. It can involve splinting of the area and even icing for seventy-two hours if any other tissues are involved.
- **Deep scar tissue work**—Break up scar tissue fibers that are not parallel.
- **Eccentric strengthening**—Organize the fibers in parallel lines.

We mentioned that the inflammation is actually somewhat of a good thing since it calls in the troops to fix the damage. But tendons don't have any inflammation and can't cry for help. We need to do something else to directly target healing in the tendon. Eccentric exercise (lengthening under contraction) actually generates a small piezoelectric current inside the tendon. This electrical charge is the stimulus to get the tendon renovation started. This needs to occur in high doses; about 40–60 reps a day for 5–6 weeks is what it takes to improve tendon strength. This is yet another example where rest will *not* improve the strength of the injured tissue.

Ligaments

A seat belt lies across your lap and your chest. You can still wiggle around and even move a bit in a seat belt, but if you try to move too far, the seat belt stops you. Ligaments function very much like a seat belt. They attach bones to bones and limit end-range mobility. While they are not drawn tight through each and every movement during running, their relative tightness around the joint helps balance tissue tension around the joints. These tough but flexible bands stabilize and guide the motion of bones. They are not capable of contraction (active shortening) but can become thicker and stronger as a positive adaptation to training. They are oriented to resist tension along a very specific direction. For the most part, they get their nutrition from fluid inside the joints and do not have a dedicated blood supply.

Ligaments are most frequently damaged through a very high strain rate such as falling or a sudden twist of a joint. This damage results in a partial micro-tear or full-thickness tear, which results in some amount of instability of the joint that the ligaments were meant to stabilize. Sprains can be graded based on the location of the joint and the ligaments' orientation. Ligament sprains typically heal to 97–98 percent of their original strength. Some ligaments, such as the medial collateral ligament (MCL) on the inside of the knee, can heal quite readily on their own, while others, such as the anterior cruciate ligament in the center of the knee, typically requires surgical intervention to repair.

Megan is trail running one Saturday morning and is in the middle of an interval. She is pretty tired and has poor foot placement on a rocky downhill. She goes down and has sharp pain in the ankle. What happened? The most frequently sprained ligament in the ankle is the anterior talofibular ligament. It runs along the outside of the ankle and is slack when the ankle is pronated (rolled inwards), and is drawn taut when the ankle is supinated (rolled out-wards). It's almost impossible to damage the anterior talofibular ligament in pronation because there is no stress on it. However, Megan's poor foot position resulted in a very quick outward roll of the foot (supination) that was enough to tear this ligament. Megan gets up and is able to finish her run with a slight limp. When she gets back to her car twenty minutes later, she notices pro-nounced swelling on the outside of the ankle. Since the tear in the ligament re-duces her ability to stabilize the ankle, her body swells to temporarily splint the area. Megan is pretty smart and ices her ankle for seventy-two hours and takes a week off from running and instead cross-trains. After a week, the swelling is reduced completely. She has no pain and decides to resume running. How does she do? We'll get back to Megan later in this chapter.

Muscle

Muscles create tension on our pulleys and levers to produce movement. Muscle is highly metabolically demanding, consuming a lot of energy both at rest and during activity. The more muscle tissue you have, the greater your caloric needs are, even at rest, to maintain your current body mass. Muscles get their blood supply from dedicated arteries. The ability of muscle tissue to actively shorten and lengthen is what distinguishes muscle from the rest of the body. Individual muscles are able to produce several hundred pounds of force to move the levers on which they insert.

The whole muscle (a), the muscle cell or fiber comprised of myofibrils (b), and the contractile unit called the sarcomere with its overlapping myosin and actin filaments, are all held together by connective tissues.

a

whole muscle

b   muscle cell
    (muscle fiber)

d

myofibril

c

sarcomere

myosin filament
actin filament

Actin and *myosin* are contractile myofilaments made of protein that lie adjacent to each other within the *sarcomere* (muscle cell). At rest, the proteins and enzymes that allow them to bond are inactive. Upon the nerve sending the signal to the muscle, calcium floods in to activate the bonding sites, allowing actin to slide over myosin. This process requires energy and causes the muscle to shorten and produce internal force. A *concentric contraction* occurs when the muscle is producing force, and the muscle is shortening. *Eccentric contractions* occur when the muscle is producing force, but the muscle is lengthening. Eccentric contractions are commonly termed "negatives" in the weight room. *Isometric contractions* occur when the muscle is generating force, but the muscle length is held constant.

Through training, muscles can generate more force. This occurs through *hypertrophy* and improvements in *nerve control*. Hypertrophy is an increase in the cross-sectional area of the muscle belly. This process takes 6–8 weeks to manifest and yields tissue that is capable of producing greater force in a single contraction. Nerve control deals more with the connection between the muscle and the brain.

Meet Sara. She has never lifted weights because her high school coach didn't "believe in it." Now in her freshman year in college, she has access to a wealth of resources such as a strength and conditioning coach. On her first day ever on squats, she is able to press 95 pounds for 8 reps. After four weeks, she has progressed to 135 pounds for 8 reps. Sara's friend comments that she has gotten stronger over the past month. Has Sara really gotten "stronger"? No. Remember that true gains in strength take 6–8 weeks and are the result of an increased cross-sectional area. It's only been four weeks, and Sara has shown considerable progress. It's no doubt that continued work in the weight room would lead to improvements in cross-sectional areas (true strength) over time, but it didn't occur within this four–week period. For the answer, we need to look to the nerves that control the muscles.

Muscle contraction is dependent on some type of input from a *motor neuron* through the *neuromuscular junction*. A *motor neuron* is a nerve fiber that tells muscles to contract. A *motor unit* is defined as the motor neuron and the muscle fibers it innervates. Muscles requiring more fine motor control have greater nerve input to the muscle fibers. Muscles in the eye require very precise control and may have as high as a 1:1 ratio of motor neurons to muscle fibers. Conversely, larger muscles such as the quadriceps may have one motor neuron innervating several hundred muscle fibers. Thus, the nervous system's hard-wiring of muscle is high when precision is the critical factor, not force.

Regardless of the ratio, the nervous system can refine its ability to control muscle. Sara's initial improvements in the ability to move weight are due to a refining of neuromuscular control. Training produces a more rapid and synchronous activation of motor units so that force can be generated more quickly to improve performance. These changes can occur rather quickly as the brain "figures out" the easiest way to control the body during the movement. Neuromuscular coordination occurs through three primary means:

1. **Number**—A single motor neuron initiates contraction of the muscle fibers it innervates. With training, the body learns to activate more motor neurons at once to recruit more muscle mass to produce more force.
2. **Frequency**—Impulses from the nerve arise faster when greater force of contraction is required (less lag time).
3. **Synchronization**—Impulses from individual nerves respond together to produce greater net activity.

The improvements in voluntary muscle control are further modified by improvements in reflex pathways. These involuntary mechanisms operate both in a *feedback* and *feed-forward* nature to adjust the state of muscle contraction.

They modify activation of the muscles to smooth and protect the body during movement. Two of the predominant mechanisms are the *Golgi tendon organ (GTO)* and *muscle spindle* fibers. GTO nerve fibers are sensitive to increased tension inside the muscle. When tension inside the muscle becomes too high, the GTO inhibits muscle contraction to limit overstrain inside the muscle. Thus the GTO operates in a *feedback* loop (increased activation = inhibition). Muscle spindles operate in a *feed-forward* loop and are responsive to changes in muscle length and velocity. Muscle spindles constantly adjust to deficiencies in length and velocity and send excitatory signals to maintain some aspect of tone within the muscle. These two mechanisms work in concert to regulate tension inside the muscle within a set window during high exertion activity. These mechanisms can be either up or downward regulated based upon the training stimulus.

To summarize, initial improvements in the ability to generate force are the result of improvements in neural control, while the long-term improvements will be a mixture of hypertrophy and neural control. Since the stance phase of running is quite short, rapid feedback from the nervous system to control joint stability and transfer force is paramount in running. Unfortunately, this is *one of the most overlooked aspects of athletic skill in runners*! Fortunately, this is very easy to identify and correct. We'll explore this more in the next chapters.

All muscle is not created the same, and thus, each responds differently to training. There are three main types of skeletal muscle fibers in every runner's body: Type I (slow twitch), Type IIX (fast-twitch glycolytic), and Type IIA (fast-twitch oxidative). Every runner has a different blend of all of these fiber types. *Mitochondria*, the cellular component responsible for aerobic metabolism, is in high concentration in Type I fibers. Since they efficiently utilize oxygen and are more resistant to fatigue, well-trained Type I fibers are the hallmark of distance runners. Type IIX fibers are capable of greater force production, but fatigue at a quicker rate. These fibers are more critical for athletes that require power development (sprinters, jumpers, throwers). Type IIA fibers are transitional and can change properties based on the type of training you do. A Type IIA fiber will never actually become a Type I or Type II, but they can become more similar. More aerobic training adapts Type IIA fibers to better utilize oxygen and resist fatigue at the expense of generating less peak force. Although all runners have all three types of fibers in their body, the distribution of each of these types is inherently genetic. Although it is possible to improve the characteristics of each muscle fiber type through training, it is not possible to alter the fiber type itself. So don't waste time wishing you had more fast-twitch muscle fibers or vice versa. It is what makes athletes unique. We all know runners who can plug along at a given pace for a 5K, and that's practically their same pace for the marathon. Their high concentration of slow-twitch fibers is efficient over the long haul, yet they just can't generate any top end speed. On the flip side, there is always someone who hangs out midpack for all but the closing stretch of the race and just blows everyone away in the last 400 meters. This person obviously has greater fast-twitch fibers.

Why don't sprinters do long runs to maintain some base level of fitness? Sprint performance is dependent on the maximal rate of force production. While long, slow runs would improve the ability of these fibers to utilize oxygen, they directly impair the ability of the sprinter to generate force. Interestingly, it takes a *significant* amount of aerobic training to get Type IIA fibers to shift closer to the characteristics of Type I fibers (better use of oxygen for energy), and it takes almost no training to get them to shift back to Type IIX fibers. That's correct—just sitting on the couch is all that it takes to keep these fibers maxed out to generate force. That is why you'll either see sprinters running fast or not at all.

A Comparison of Muscle Fiber Types

Feature	Type I Red slow-twitch (fatigue-resistant)	Type IIA Intermediate fast-twitch	Type IIX White fast-twitch (fatigable)
Metabolic Characteristics			
Twitch rate	Slow	Fast	Fast
Myosin ATPase activity	Slow	Fast	Fast
ATP synthesis pathway	Aerobic	Aerobic	Anaerobic
Myoglobin content	High	High	Low
Glycogen stores	Low	Intermediate	High
Rate of fatigue	Slow	Intermediate	Fast
Structural Characteristics			
Color	Red	Red (pink)	White (pale)
Fiber diameter	Small	Intermediate	Large
Mitochondria	Many	Many	Few
Capillaries	Many	Many	Few

Since you can't realistically change your dominant fiber type, don't stress. Instead, tailor your individual training towards optimizing the properties of our fiber types for the events in which you compete. For those wanting to now exactly what percentage of fiber types you have, it is possible, but it's ainful. If you *really* want to know, you can get a muscle biopsy. A nice scienist essentially takes a core sample of your belly and then sends it off to the ab for analysis. But in all honesty, what would this really tell you? You can't hange it. Oh, one more thing. Women—you are in control here. That's right— he genetic code regulating your mitochondria (ability to use oxygen) is based n your mother's DNA, not your proud Poppa's. So Dad, little junior or junior-tte won't care if you got a medal in the Olympics. Your biggest challenge is naking sure that Mom got one.

The position of the muscle has a profound impact on its ability to produce orce. This is termed the *length-tension relationship* of a muscle. In a perfect vorld, the actin and myosin filaments would always be in a perfect amount of ension for optimal contraction. However, muscles change in length as the joint hanges position. There is a bell-shaped curve of force production that depends n the length of the muscle.

To demonstrate this concept, make a tight fist. Squeeze it as hard as you an. Now, while keeping your fist as tight as you can, flex your wrist forward so hat it comes closer to the front side of your forearm. Notice that it's impos-ible to keep the fist as tight. The muscles that tense the fist have become

Length-Tension Relationship

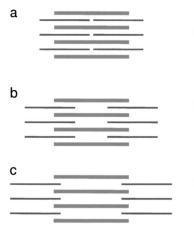

a. *Overly flexed joints have too much overlap between actin (thin line) and myosin (thick line), making it tough to further shorten the muscle for rapid energy production.*

b. *A mild amount of flex in a joint allows the muscles to shorten slightly and otimizes the amount of overlap between fibers for rapid force production.*

c. *Too much straightening of the joint lengthens the individual fibers and makes it harder to rapidly shorten the muscle.*

Locked limbs prevent your muscles from entering their optimal length-tension window.

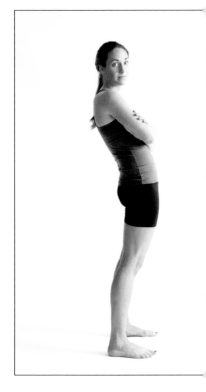

overly shortened and produce less force. Keeping your fist tight, return your wrist to its neutral position and notice that your fist becomes stronger. You are now in the optimal window. Finally, keeping the wrist as tight as you can, extend your wrist all the way back and notice that the grip strength is yet again decreased—this time due to over-lengthening.

What does this have to do with the legs or running? Stand up and prepare to jump up for maximum vertical height. Do this once or twice and get some sense of how challenging it is. Now, squat all the way down as low as you can go, and repeat the jump. Think about your jump performance in light of the length-tension relationship. Prior to your initial jump, you naturally bent all the joints in the legs to pre-tension the muscles and place the actin and myosin filaments in their optimal position. In the full squat, the filaments were overly lengthened, taking additional time and effort to raise the body's center of mass. Think about the start of your 5K. Do you stand straight with knees locked or drop down into a full squat prior to the gun? No. You crouch slightly to prepare for an efficient takeoff. This same flexed-limb "ready position" is utilized to optimize the length-tension relationship in field sports, tennis, basketball, etc.

Like other tissues in the body, muscle has a certain amount of elasticity that allows it to expand to a given length and then return to its resting length. The amount of elongation a muscle is able to undergo is dependent on its:

1. **Flexibility**—The arrangement of muscle fibers is similar to a bunch of straws bundled together. Individual muscle cells (called sarcomeres) line up end to end within the tube to form a muscle fiber. To use an analogy, a layer of plastic wrap (connective tissue) binds the tubes (muscle fibers) together into *muscle fascicles*. Yet another layer of plastic wrap

binds these muscle fascicles into what we think of as muscles. How does this impact flexibility? The "tubes" themselves will shorten or lengthen as the muscle contracts. But if the plastic wrap is too tight, it limits the normal shortening and lengthening of the fibers, restricting total muscle length. While it is possible to improve flexibility, there are limitations imposed by genetics. The plastic wrap in some runners can be generically supertight or superloose compared to the norm. These folks can change, but they may be shifted so far to the outside that they'll never be in the middle of the pack. And this is OK! People are different. Age is another factor. As we age, structures stiffen and lose their ability to elongate. Improvements in flexibility come from *long duration* stretches that *physically tear* the tissue surrounding muscle fibers to increase mobility within the muscle.

2. **Neural Stiffness**—Muscle structure has a certain amount of internal tension. Some of this tension is based on the orientation of the connective tissue mentioned above, and some of this stiffness is the result of neural control (muscle spindle and golgi tendon organ reflex loops). Since stiffness is defined as the resistance to a change in length, a runner with greater stiffness would have a slightly higher level of baselevel muscle contraction at a quiet state as compared to a runner with less stiffness. Having a nervous system with greater stiffness is actually a good thing for some athletes. Stiffer muscles better transfer forces to the tendon instead of absorbing forces inside the muscle. This is something you can actually improve, and we'll discuss it in Chapter 6.

Cartilage

Where two or more bones come together, we find a joint. The ligaments that surround and stabilize the joint typically blend together to form a *capsule* (imagine a Ziploc bag) that creates a closed environment around the joint space. The ends of these bones are covered in a material called *cartilage*, which provides shock absorption and decreases friction between the joint surfaces. Bone on bone contact is not good. Since there is no blood supply to the inside of the joint, cartilage receives its nutrition from *synovial fluid* that lies within the joint. This fluid is pumped about through normal movement to lubricate and nourish the cartilage surface.

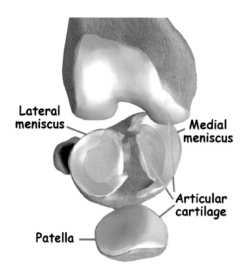

Lateral meniscus

Medial meniscus

Articular cartilage

Patella

Healthy cartilage covering the joint surfaces keeps your parts gliding nicely.

When soccer mom pulls up to pick up her kids from practice, you can easily see the minivan door opening up. What you can't see is the more complex movement of the parts inside the door. This is similar to our anatomy. While we obviously see big movements—a shoulder reaching overhead, a knee extending straight—there is also very specific motion that occurs on the joint surfaces. This roll, spin, and glide that occurs between the bones creates compression, tension, and shear forces. Cartilage is able to respond well to compression and decompression, and less so to shear forces. Higher rates of loading (either more force or force applied too quickly) further stress the integrity of cartilage.

The alignment of the bones, the muscles, tendons, and ligaments is critical to pressure exerted on the surfaces of the joints. Imagine a door pivoting around its hinge. The hinge has a specific axis of rotation and can tolerate millions of cycles of opening and closing without a problem. Now imagine twisting the door while swinging it open and closed. The addition of the twisting force creates excessive shear forces on the hinges and accelerates their wear. The goal is to keep the joint in its respective alignment.

Different runners have different structural alignment and will move differently while running. Have you ever seen a runner run excessively "toe out" or "duck-footed"? Have you ever told that person to point their feet straight? It's probably better to keep your mouth shut in this situation. There are a number of reasons why a runner might point his or her feet outwards when running. If their toe-out is simply due to habit or muscular tightness, then it should be addressed and corrected. However, this toe-out pattern may be due to their skeletal alignment. Let's say the runner has an externally rotated tibia (lower leg) that causes his feet to point out. If he runs this way, he keeps his knee alignment in check and will likely go on for many more miles. If you told this person to point his feet straight, he would force the knee into excessive internal rotation throughout the run cycle. Over time, this would increase contact on areas of the joint that were not designed to tolerate such high loads and accelerate shear across the joint surface. Telling this runner to point his feet straight would *increase* their risk of developing knee pain, shin splints, and an ACL tear. And you thought you were being helpful! Clinical evaluation of the runner's femoral anteversion/retroversion and tibial torsion dictates the rotational limb position that they should maintain throughout their gait. If you are not skilled in these terms or how to evaluate them, refrain from imposing your preconceptions and refer them to someone who is. The goal of running is to keep one's dynamic alignment in check with your structural alignment. Everyone is aligned slightly differently and that's 100 percent OK, as long as each runner can maintain his individual alignment as he runs.

Individuals who don't possess enough dynamic muscular control to maintain *their* structural alignment during running are subject to premature wear of the cartilage. The best cartilage is called *hyaline* cartilage. This stuff is golden. Quite simply it does the best job at dispersing the load at the joint surface. Abnormal shear as a result of instability, poor alignment, or excessive activity results in wearing away of this essential layer. Cartilage has no pain sensation. It is not until this hyaline layer is completely worn away that there is bone on bone contact and pain fibers that alert you to the damage that has been caused. Well, that stinks, right? Let's look at how this typically plays out.

So you go to the doctor. Your joint hurts. You've been told you have mild arthritis and you sulk; your running career is over; you are doomed; the sky is falling. All too often, patients tell me, "Well, I used to do ____, but then I got arthritis and stopped." Guess what. Osteoarthritis is simply inflammation in the joint space. With the cartilage layer gone, the excessive shearing of bone on bone causes pain and inflammation. What should you do? Specifically, do you have to stop running? It depends. Let's look a bit deeper at what causes this excessive wear and tear at the joint.

The joint surfaces are capable of withstanding numerous cycles of repetitive motion. (Trillions? Zillions?) A door can open and shut forever as long as the motion occurs through the axis of the hinge and someone remembers to oil that hinge once in a while. Well, the synovial fluid can lube your body's hinges, but if your muscles don't control the slop in the joint, this rotational axis shifts. It's as if someone is "twisting" the door as it moves through the range. The joint surfaces are now being loaded in a way in which they were not designed and cannot tolerate. And things get bad. Most problems in overuse injury result from an inability to stabilize the rotational and frontal plane alignment of the joint as it moves though a normal path. Gee, have you read this somewhere already in this book? Think this point might be *really* important? It is because your hyaline cartilage in that location is gone forever. Yes, if it is unloaded enough, a similar tissue called *fibrocartilage* will grow back to take its place. While this is certainly better than nothing at all, it has a reduced durability and ability to distribute load at the joint surface.

So what should you do? Don't wait around for an inferior cartilage tissue to come to your rescue. If the problem was abnormal joint contact due to poor alignment, let's shift focus back to correcting the dynamic alignment! If you correct your ability to control the slop in the joint so that the motion now occurs around the normal axis of the joint, you put the majority of the load *back to where it should be*. This is the long-term solution for dealing with degeneration in the joint surfaces. Examination of these suspect mechanics will be covered in following chapters, although if you are someone who has been told they fall into this category, you should seek professional help. Find a physical therapist who is well known in your area for dealing with runners and sports injuries. You want to keep your own parts as long as possible. So arthritis doesn't mean your career is over unless you see your doc and he tells you that you have pretty significant narrowing of the space inside the joint. This is less promising. It's not 100 percent the end of the world (exceptions—I have had a few patients who have been told this and they continue to run ultramarathons), but it means that the joint itself is less able to tolerate the loads you see in running and anything else you like to do. The joint likely won't tolerate lots of high-load activity. Maybe it's time to buy a bike for at least a portion of your miles or more. But you can still do a better job of aligning your parts. Indentify why you aren't loading the joint correctly and fix it so that the stress goes back to the right place within the joint.

So we need to address one final white elephant in the room. You say "Doc, it hurts when I run." He tells you to stop or you'll wreck your joints. How many health care providers and friends have told you this? I stopped counting a long time ago. So let's look at this head-on: Is running bad for cartilage? Does it cause osteoarthritis (degenerative changes in the joint)? Let's take a cursory look at the literature. The research on cartilage is composed of lab studies, animal studies, and human studies. None of them are all-inclusive or perfectly designed, but let's summarize the findings. The existing literature does not reveal a clear causative relationship between distance running and joint health for those running a low volume less than twenty-five miles per week. The literature does reveal increased incidence of degenerative findings on imaging (X-ray, MRI, CT Scan) for those running more than sixty-five miles per week; however, there is little correlation among degenerative findings on imaging and pain. Thus, while you may have degenerative changes in the joint, you may have no pain at all. And you may have pain with little to no degenerative changes within the joint. The highest incidence of arthritis is found in individuals who have a history of heavy lifting and bending, such a factory workers.

The normal mechanism for providing nutrition for cartilage is compression, decompression, and gliding. These all occur during running. It appears that *some amount* of running is actually good for joints to stimulate remodeling. *More* than that is even better, and more than that is actually worse. No one really knows where the limit is on this from a population standpoint, let alone a personal one. From a professional opinion, it would be tough to make the case that running fifty marathons in a year would be a healthy undertaking. For the vast majority of runners, this would result in both short- and long-term stress on the joint surface. However, there are numerous individuals who perform feats like this each and every year, without injury. Perhaps (hopefully!) they have excellent joint alignment and exceptional neuromuscular stabilization to keep their body dynamically aligned. Mild to moderate running volume appears to be a healthy stimulus for the long-term maintenance of cartilage. Evidence suggests that some activity (running) is better for joint surfaces than no activity (not running). Maybe it's time to ask the naysayers if they want to join you for a run . . .

Charlie is a typical middle-aged runner, highly active in many endurance sports. Over time, he's developed knee pain. His doctor tells him that he's created a meniscal tear and the loose flap that is floating around and creating pain should be removed. Mike has surgery and within five to six days is pain-free and returns to running. So is this the end of the story? Unfortunately, no.

When the meniscus it torn or removed, incidence of early onset arthritis increases at an alarming rate. Why? Your meniscus has a job—it helps distribute pressure across the joint surface and provides mechanical stability at the knee. The mechanical support provided by the meniscus helps provide a barrier to the "neutral zone" that the muscles around the knee must stabilize. With a defect in the meniscus, the end range barrier is gone, and there is more potential "slop" within the joint. If uncontrolled, this slop leads to accelerated breakdown of cartilage.

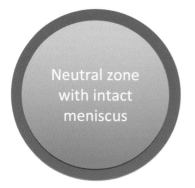

Neutral zone with intact meniscus

Increased neutral zone with meniscus damage

The green circle on the left represents the mechanical restraint of an intact meniscus. Muscles normally stabilize the zone shaded in blue. On the right is Charlie's knee. With the medial meniscus gone, there is less mechanical stability present and an increased demand for muscular control to maintain health of the joint surfaces. The good news is that Charlie's current MRI shows no significant breakdown at the joint at this time. If he stays on top of his knee stability, he should be able to continue running with a significantly reduced risk for arthritis over the long term. A smart training plan goes beyond long runs and speed work. It addresses all your unique biomechanical needs to ensure that you are racking up miles well into the future.

The Musculoskeletal System

Most of this chapter was spent identifying why parts are different. Understanding these differences is critical. However, the body can't work with just one of those parts; it works together as a system. So let's unite this discussion by checking back in with Megan, our poor runner who sprained her ankle but got right back up and continued running. Over the next six months she notices that she now "rolls" this ankle more than she used to, and on a few occasions she even has minor swelling following one of these events. Megan is now someone we define as having *chronic ankle instability*. Considering ligaments heal to 97–98 percent of original strength, why does Megan's ligament tear result in chronic problems?

Obviously the body is designed to move. It can move around in lots of different ways because you have a certain amount of accessory motion or "slop" in every joint. If you didn't have slop then you could only move in one way. Enough slop allows swimmers, gymnasts, power lifters, skateboarders, and runners to move in different ways. However, we need to control this slop to keep all our parts working together. This is called *stability*, and it's not something that just happens passively.

The stability of the body is made up of the bones and joints that provide structure, the ligaments that provide some type of end-range restraint at the joint, and the muscles and tendons that produce movement. All of these parts are different yet "talk" to each other and coordinate movement via the nervous system. These nerves allow for *proprioception*, or the ability to "sense" the position of a joint without looking at it.

Most of these nerves that provide us with a sense of our joint position are within the intact ligaments themselves. So when Megan tore her ligament, the imbedded nerves were torn as well. While the ligament is capable of healing back to almost full strength, these nerves don't regenerate (even if a surgical repair of the ligament is performed). So while the mechanical function of the ligament is restored, the neural feedback to the brain is permanently altered. During the acute injury, structure was damaged, and the body swelled enough to say, "Hey, Megan—take it easy on us—we are hurt!" As swelling goes away, we feel as if we recovered and train as if we recovered, all with less input from the nerves. This diminished input means that Megan has a hard time stabilizing the slop in her ankle even though the physical structure of the ligament is pretty well healed. This lack of control makes us more likely to injure the area again, as indicated by Megan's minor sprains and swelling during running.

So should she stop running? No way—she should take steps to fix the weak link in the chain. Fortunately, the brain has redundancy, or multiple ways of getting feedback to sense joint position. Other parts of the system will step up when other parts are down and out. Megan begins balance and proprioception training to improve the fine motor coordination of her foot and ankle muscles

Rest doesn't fix problems. What does it do in each tissue?

Bone	Weakens collagen structure and mineral density
Capsule	Shrinks it, increases resistance to movement
Ligament	Decreases cross-links, decreases tensile strength
Tendon	Disorganizes collagen, decreases tensile strength
Muscle	Decreases contractile proteins
Cartilage	Causes swelling and weakens binding agents

Since none of those sound like good things, how do you improve each tissue?

Bone	Slight increase in compression/vibration to increase mineral density and strength
Capsule	Mobilization through activity in the physiologic range with manual work if needed
Ligament	Progressive tensile stress in the line of force (loading as much a you can under controlled conditions)
Tendon	Progressive eccentric strengthening to improve the organization of collagen fibers – goal to improve strain distribution and strength
Muscle	Low-load exercise to induce metabolic adaptations, then alter speed and force of contraction to recruit different motor units
Cartilage	Moderate loads through available ROM

to improve the input back to the brain and close the gap on her deficits. Rehabilitation from ligament sprains should always include proprioception training to ensure that both mechanical and proprioceptive functions are optimized. We'll cover more on this in Chapter 7.

Summary

- Your body's musculoskeletal system is made of various parts.
- While the system functions as a whole, the different tissues of the system break down and rebuild at different rates in response to training.
- Rest helps calm down acute inflammatory events but does not result in any type of positive tissue adaptation.
- Individual parts coordinate and communicate via the nervous system.
- Injury to the mechanical parts will impair this coordination and produce an unstable body segment. This can be improved via specific training that goes beyond just more miles per week.

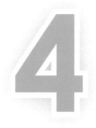

Beyond the Mileage Log— There's More to It Than Running Hard Runs and Long Runs

You: Hey—can you take a look at my car? It's making a funny noise, and it's not that fast.

Mechanic: Sure—how many miles are on it?

You: About 73,000.

Mechanic: What kind of maintenance have you done over the car's life?

You: Nothing.

Mechanic: Ummmm . . . no oil changes? Timing belt checks? Filters? Tires?

You: Nope. I just park it in the garage and expect it to go without any issues when needed.

Mechanic: Ummm. Ahhh. Riiiiight. Well . . . (sigh) let's take a look then.

If we rewrote this screenplay with your name in lights, you'd likely feel pretty stupid, or careless, or regretful, or some combination thereof. It's sort of understood that the things we own and use often are subject to wear and tear, and require periodic maintenance to stay in top shape. We won't point any fingers, but let's change the word "car" above to "body." Change "mechanic" to "Doc." And most likely change "73,000 miles" to some number much lower. If you aren't putting these things together, I'll just go ahead and ask: Your body has parts—what specific things are you doing on a routine basis to make sure they perform as intended? Deafening . . . radio . . . silence . . . Does anyone actually hear the pin drop? Hello?

The million dollar question: "What's the best way to run and am I doing it?" I get asked this every day. Some folks claim that runners will "find" their optimal biomechanical economy through training. They think running longer and faster is always the answer to running better. Is it possible to say that all the higher mileage runners are more efficient than the lower mileage runners? The literature does support the idea that a group of high mileage runners tends to be more economical than a group of runners who run less mileage. More experienced runners are better at transferring elastic energy in their bodies. Practice makes perfect, right? So it is true: the more you run, the better you should become at running. However, this research focuses on groups of runners, and not the individual runner.

Everyone has different ingredients, and your casserole is only as good as the ingredients *you* throw in it. Your bone length, alignment, soft tissue mobility, muscular stability, strength, speed, and movement skills all wind up in a plug-and-play scenario. It is likely that you have figured out the "best" way to run with your current attributes, but what if the white elephant in the room is actually your body? Muscle imbalances and mobility restrictions introduce flaws into a runner's gait that are typically greater than the sum of the individual parts. Where would the performance ceiling bump up to? We can't define optimal gait until we've identified optimal ingredients. Good ingredients equal good food.

The second most asked question is: "How do I compare to (insert idol/ nemesis here)?" Should you try to model the running form of the current record

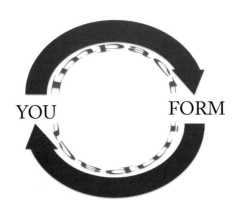

YOU   FORM

holder in the event of your choice? There are no well-controlled studies to support the idea that all runners should run the same way all the time. There is lots of variability in running form, and there is nothing inherently bad about that. My experience has been somewhat unique. In my lab, I obtain stacks of graphs of various biomechanical parameters for each and every runner I see. Each and every evaluation is its own ministudy and has given me a unique perspective on efficiency.

I'd agree that higher mileage runners in general tend to be more efficient on the whole, but not entirely so. Some of the most efficient forms (mechanical work/metabolic work) I've measured have been moms with four kids. However, the combination of low physiologic potential (bad genes) and the stress of taking care of four kids limits the woman's ability to perform. I've seen world-caliber athletes that are very lucky since they have big engines, but subpar form. The most beautiful data set I've ever laid eyes on belonged to a sub-30-minute 10K runner. Now sub-30 is something to be proud of, but it's not going to win you a medal at World's. Additionally, there is no research to show that elite runners sustain less injury than low mileage runners.

What does this mean? Like Mom said, "Don't stereotype people you meet." Each individual should be looked at separately. The style of an individual's running *does* affect the stress the body sees when running. The goal is to optimize the combination of dynamic stability, soft tissue mobility, and running form to produce the most efficient runner.

And lastly, what are your goals? Before anyone can say what is the best way to run, you have to come to terms with why you run and what running means to you. Running for fitness at an easy pace is a great way to stay healthy for the long term. It does require certain attributes from you, but at a lower threshold. On the flip side, if your goal is to beat your personal record (PR) at all costs, it's also fairly easy to describe how you should run. While there is no research to show that running fast is hurtful, it requires *more mobility* and *more force*. Do you have it? Because if you don't, your fast form is going to set you up for overuse injury and compromised efficiency. If you want to crank up the pace, *you have to earn it.*

Step 1. Optimize the body.

Step 2. Optimize your form.

Guess who is in charge of the body mentioned in Step 1. You are. Scary, isn't it?

Great athletes are always working on their weakest link. This book centers around identifying and correcting factors that are unique to you. Improving the chassis allows you to optimize your horsepower. The tests in this book were specifically chosen as they have the biggest impact on form, injury prevention, and economy in runners. I have access to one of the nicest gait labs in the country that tells me exactly what each and every runner is doing. However, I still perform these tests on each and every runner I see. Why? Because you'll never know why someone moves the way they do until you evaluate it. Hey, you! Simply reading through the tests won't help; do the test and follow the plan. Improving your results will ultimately provide new skills that directly translate into your running.

It's time to take all this conceptual background knowledge and make some sense out of how it impacts the way you move, the strength you generate, and the way you run. This information in the applied chapters section will provide evidence of the need to make a change. I'm all for opinions, and no one has all the answers for everyone all the time, but before you form an opinion, it's probably useful to know the science, even if those facts run against the lore handed down over the years. Let's put less emphasis on tradition and more emphasis on what makes sense. Remember the injury rates of 82 percent? This is a number we are trying to bring down.

Range of Motion: Enough is Enough

The range of motion required to run is more constrained, and much smaller than say, for a gymnast. The majority of the motion occurs in one single plane. If we have enough mobility to move at each and every joint for the motion required to run then there really isn't much of a problem. However, runners that lack motion in specific areas: A) move more from somewhere else to make up the difference, B) alter their gait mechanics, or C) both. These compensations create imbalances in tissue stress over the long term.

Roundabouts and Restrictions

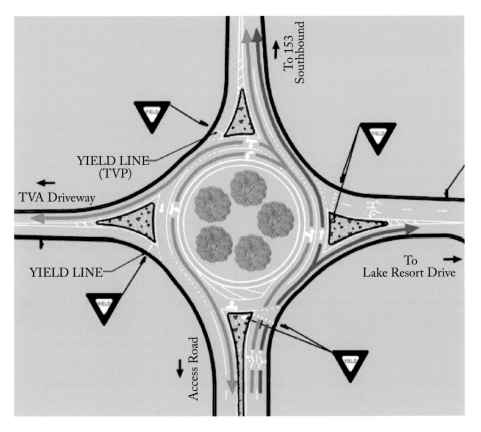

If you can't go straight, you have to increase motion in another plane.

Imagine running straight down the road and reaching a four-way intersection. What's the path of least resistance through the intersection? Straight through, right? Yes! Let's apply this to the ankle joint. You are running straight ahead. If you have adequate dorsiflexion in the sagittal plane, the lower leg can roll over the foot smoothly during the stance phase. The dominant path of the joint and the runner remain in the sagittal plane.

After half a mile, you reach the next intersection. This time it's one of those European-inspired roundabouts. You can't move straight through the intersection this time and are forced to rotate around the circle. Let's go back to the ankle. During the propulsion phase, the ankle needs to roll over the foot to move the body past the contact point. If the runner has limited dorsiflexion mobility in the sagittal plane, it will increase motion in another plane to get the center of mass past the foot. Oftentimes the runner will compensate by "spinning" off the forefoot during push-off (this is referred to as a "whip"). Limited motion in one joint increases out-of-plane motion in another. Excessive out-of-plane mobility increases demand on muscles and is a major risk factor for injury.

Strength: How Much Does a Runner Really Need?

Sometimes we make stupid decisions. Those decisions result in us doing dumb things. Think of your runner's body as a canoe. A canoe can support a certain amount of weight and is more stable from front to back than it is from side to side. However, it's not the most stable thing. It rocks about in all directions somewhat when you paddle in rough waters or gets really unstable if you decide to stand up. What would happen if you did something really dumb . . . like fire a cannon out of the canoe? All that force from the cannon is going to send your canoe, the cannon, and you into the water in a fraction of a second. If, in fact, you did have the need to engage in sea combat, it would be a smart decision to build some type of outrigger to stabilize the canoe if you were going to have to fire a cannon from it. It's obvious that the force from the cannon is going to compromise the stability of your canoe, and you should have prepared your vessel for it in the first place. Right now, you are probably thinking that the person in this story is an idiot.

Force and Stability

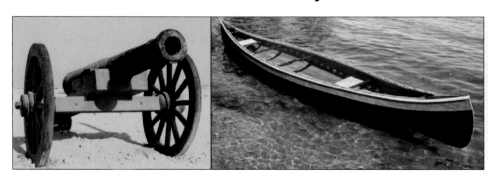

Don't fire a cannon from a canoe. High forces require a stable base of support. If the neuromuscular system fails to coordinate a stable foundation, the high forces of running are likely to create injury, impair economy, or both.

I'd hold the name calling for now though, because this person is not too far off from your typical runner. Runners run a lot. They move over and over again in a very constrained movement pattern. In fact, I have never seen a runner who has weak quads, hamstrings, and calves. These muscles are the ones that move us forward and they get some amount of strength development as you keep running in one plane over and over again . . . until 82 percent of you get hurt, or until you reach the ceiling of your performance and wonder why your times aren't improving.

Running is just a bunch of single leg squats with a flight phase in between. Not only do you have to move the body forward, but you have to lift it up and stabilize it laterally. And since stance times in distance running are between 0.15–0.25 seconds, you have to do this very, very quickly. Each time you land, you are basically falling from the sky and touching down with a force that is much higher than just your body weight. And this force doesn't just act on you from one side. It's trying to sink your "canoe" with 250 percent of your body weight, tipping it forward and back with 50 percent of your body weight, and trying to tip you over sideways with 20 percent of your body weight. When running, you have forces acting on you from *multiple planes*. Muscular strength to stabilize and counter this force is critical.

So running requires large amounts of force to keep your body stable in *multiple planes*. Since I sure put a lot of time into making good decisions about your training program to promote comprehensive athletic skills, I'll put forth the following question: What specific *multiplane* exercises and drills are you doing as part of your training program? Please list the exercises that you are doing to improve the rotational and lateral stability of the core, hips, and foot. If you can't pick up a pen and write them down instantly, let's look at what happens if you don't have dynamic strength, because I'd like to help you make better decisions and avoid an uncontrolled fall into the 82 percent of you who get hurt while doing a sport that you love.

Power is Nothing Without Control

Years of dealing with overuse injury in endurance athletes has shifted my mind-set. I'm focused on the imbalances, not the symptoms. It's not because I don't care; it's because I've learned that imbalances are present well before symptoms present themselves, and that one imbalance can lead to a variety

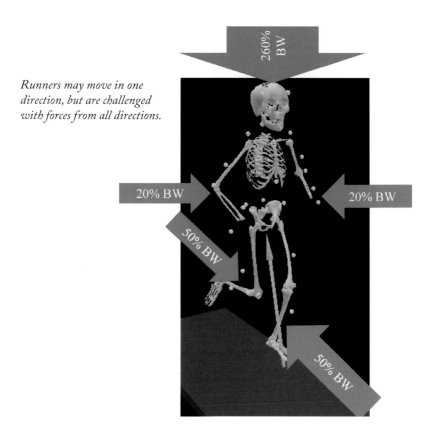

Runners may move in one direction, but are challenged with forces from all directions.

of symptoms. Achilles tendinopathy, metatarsal stress fractures, chronic ankle sprains, and shin splints all stem from the same basic movement imbalance. Wouldn't it be nice to decrease your chance of getting a bunch of injuries by addressing a few simple issues? Improving stability in the stance phase is the critical factor in staying healthy and performing at your prime.

This is not to say you should ignore your symptoms. Go see your health care provider for help here. They'll help pinpoint and stage the severity of the injury to direct you on the best course of action for right now. But if you don't dedicate some time to improve the mechanism that got you here in the first place, you are going to be calling for an office visit for the same thing sometime in the future. A smarter body can avoid getting hurt in the first place.

Summary

- "Correct" running form is dependent on the athlete's mobility, stability, and power.
- Don't emulate your best friend; emulate your best you.
- It's critical to have enough length to run.
- Proper stability and control are essential to preserving alignment, minimizing fatigue, and ensuring that high levels of force can be generated.

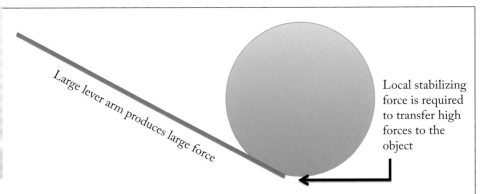

Local stabilizing force is required to transfer high forces to the object

"Give me a lever long enough and I'll move the world." We've all heard this quote, but is leverage all you need? Let's pretend you are trying to uproot a tree stump. You take your huge pry bar and stick one end under the stump. Next you push down on that lever as hard as you can. Except instead of all that force popping the stump up, the pry bar just slides to the side. Why was your effort wasted? The end of the bar wasn't braced well on the ground. Without proximal stability, you can't effectively move mountains; or the world; or your body. Every joint in the body requires coordinated muscular stability so that the primary movers can transfer high forces through your levers (bones) to run efficiently.

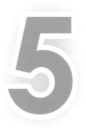

Soft Tissue Mobility—Did Gumby Have It Right?

Last year at a national conference, I attended a lecture on stretching. This lecture didn't really say anything new from a clinical perspective, but it addressed things that the fitness industry and media spin to us daily: "Stretching helps you recover faster. Stretching speeds the removal of the body's toxins. (What is a toxin anyway? It's funny that people are scared of things that don't exist!) Daily stretching results in long, lean muscles. Stretching prevents injuries." While all of these things sound great, *they just aren't true*. Having more flexibility than you need for the mechanics of running provides no advantage. In fact, it can create problems.

This statement might have thrown a good bit of you for a loop, and we'll hit more detail later. But you know what is really funny? The next day, there was a benefit 5K race before the conference. So about ten minutes prior to race start, some guy gets on the mic and blabbers: "Dr. Whatever is going to lead us through a prerun stretching routine." Umm . . . Excuse me . . . Weren't these all of the same people who were at the talk the day prior that said stretching isn't necessary for everyone? It's kind of ironic that the sport of running is "stuck in a rut." In a funny sequence of events, someone said— *"Hey, wait, why are we doing this?"* —and then the announcer (who was a doctor) said, "Good point. OK—forget it! Five minutes till race start!" The five-minute prerun stretch has become ritualistic. Do runners even need to stretch? And what happens when we stretch anyway? Or is there something else we should be focused on?

Defining Mobility

Let's define some terms so we are on the same page with how we define movement. There are three primary planes of motion: *sagittal, frontal,* and *transverse*. Since you are likely sitting while reading this book, extend your knee out in front of you and then flex it back. This is motion in the sagittal plane. Now take that same leg and move it out to the side away from your midline— this motion is in the frontal plane. Lastly, bring the leg back in line with the body and straighten your knee. While keeping the knee extended, rotate your hip so that your kneecap points outwards and then inwards. The following pictures illustrate these body movements.

Sagittal plane   **Frontal Plane**   **Transverse Plane**

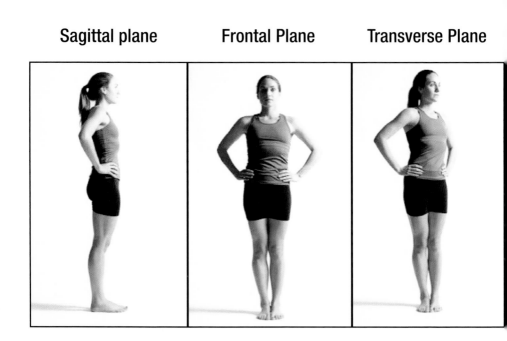

We also have terms to discuss specific motions at each joint. The following pictures illustrate movement of the joints in the lower body.

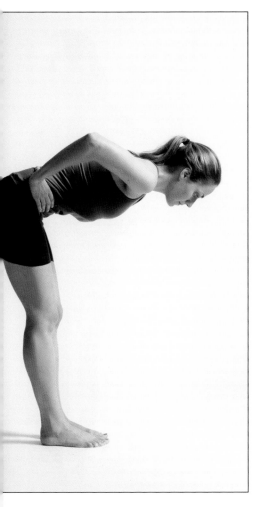

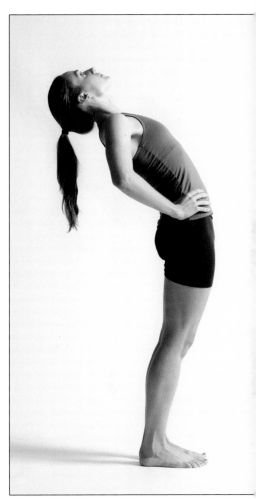

Spine flexion   Spine extension

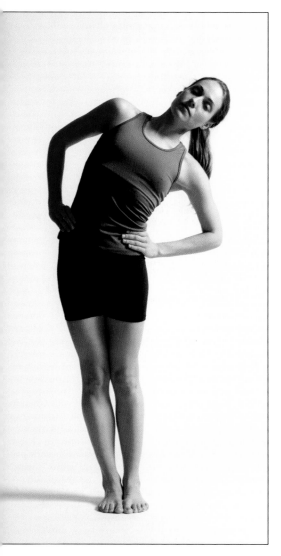

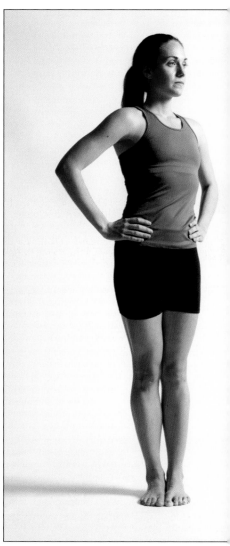

Spine side bending   Spine rotation

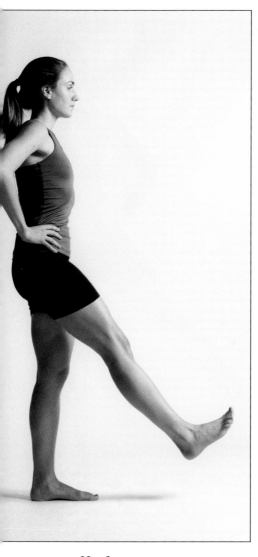

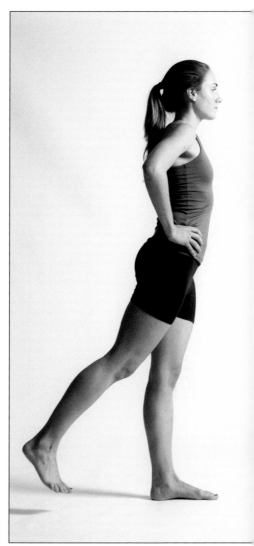

Hip flex   Hip extension

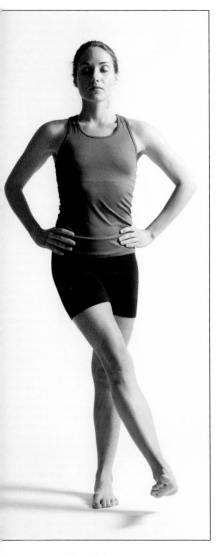

Hip adduction

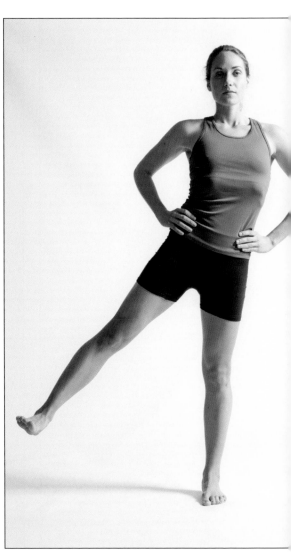

Hip abduction

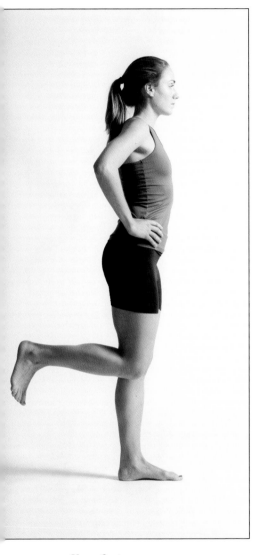

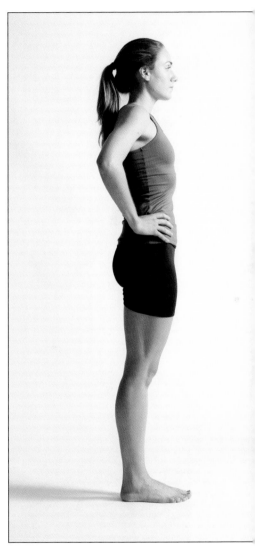

Knee flexion   Knee extension

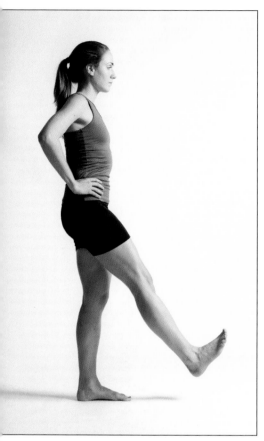

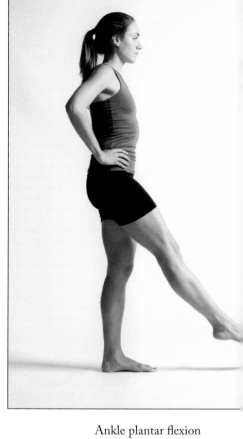

Ankle dorsiflexion

Ankle plantar flexion

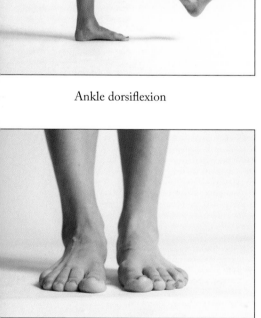

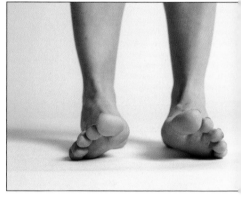

Foot pronation

Foot supination

What Types of Things Limit Mobility at a Joint?

Tissue mobility is not always the same thing as flexibility. As you now know, there is more to it than just muscle length. Gross limitations in mobility can be due to multiple factors. We are going to break up our discussion on *tissue mobility* into three aspects:

1. **Motion at the joint surface**—Are the bones *rolling, gliding,* and *spinning* on each other?
2. **Musculotendinous length**—Are tissues *long enough to allow normal movement?*
3. **Musculotendinous glide**—Are the layers *mobile enough to function normally?*

Joint Surface Mobility

Each joint has a very specific motion pattern that is dependent on the shape of the joint surfaces and the capsule that surrounds the joint. This capsule is similar to a bag and is made up of the surrounding ligaments, tendons, and fascia. The joint capsule provides structural restraint and guides the motion

Joint Surface Mobility

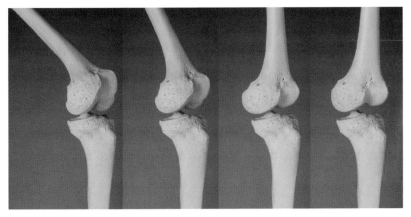

While most runners think the knee is a hinge joint, there is more going on inside than you see outside. As the knee moves, it rolls, glides, and spins. Note how the front of the femur glides back as the knee extends

that occurs at the joint surface itself. Remember, when you move a limb, there is a very specific pattern of roll, spin, and glide that occurs at each joint surface. If the capsule is too tight, it changes the axis of motion. Now the roll, spin, and glide of the joint occur in places that were never designed to tolerate this load. This increases compression and shear in the joint and causes premature wear and tear of the joint surfaces.

Moving a joint in a manner that does not use its normal contact point is the exact mechanism for developing arthritis. So if the primary limitation in joint mobility is due to a restriction in the joint capsule, the joint capsule must be mobilized in very specific directions. Once the capsular mobility is restored, the roll, spin, and glide in the joint occurs at its intended location, typically with improvement in function and elimination of pain. This is typically something you'll need to seek outside help for, as joint mobilizations are very specific and require skilled clinical hands.

When to Call for Professional Help

While limited tissue mobility of the muscle and tendon are the usual suspects that limit mobility, there are others that play a significant role. How do you know if more than just stretching is needed? Stretching should not hurt and it should provide results. If it doesn't feel like you can actually stretch what you are trying to, there may be something else going on. For example, when stretching the Achilles, gastrocnemius, and soleus (the heel chords), you should feel some tension in the *back of the calf*. If instead you feel like you are "blocked" or simply mashing the *front* of the ankle joint together, the mobility limitation is in the joint, and not the muscle and tendon. Limitations in capsular and joint surface mobility *cannot* be improved by stretching. They shift the axis of the joint away from its natural location, alter stress on the bones and cartilage, and can cause premature wear and degeneration. Correction requires specific joint mobilizations by your physical therapist to restore proper roll, glide, and spin at the joint surface. Trying to stretch into a joint restriction can actually make this worse sometimes due to increased compression inside the joint. If you feel like your efforts to improve mobility are going nowhere, seek professional help!

Tissue Length versus Tissue Stiffness versus Tissue Glide

Assuming the joint surface motion is clear, let's shift our focus to the mobility of the muscle-tendon unit. This structure has the greatest change in length during movement and thus the highest amount of strain (change in length with a given load). *Tissue glide* is much different, and I'll argue, more important for endurance athletes.

Tissue Length

Muscles and tendons have more change in length than any other tissues as we move about. If they are restricted, they shift stresses inside the joint and can cause premature breakdown. If you don't have enough range to run, they'll introduce compensations into your stride. Enough mobility to run is all you need. The idea that more is always better doesn't apply to running. There is no research to show that "extra" mobility at the joint can protect you from injury or improve your performance.

So what does stretching actually do to your body? Webster's online dictionary defines stretching as: *To make longer in length; to enlarge or distend, especially by force; to cause the limbs of a person to be pulled, especially in torture.* Translation: Stretching literally rips apart collagen bonds of the connective tissues in the musculoskeletal system. Destroying these bonds loosens the structure and results in increased length.

All this tearing has an upside and a downside. Tearing structures actually creates an inflammatory event and impairs the body's ability to perform at peak capacity. This is why "everyone stretching everything all the time" is pretty much a bad idea. We don't want to create inflammation and promote swelling in training athletes. If you have enough mobility to run, there is no logical rationale to stretch. No one has ever shown more tissue length than required for a specific sport to be beneficial for either performance or injury. However, if a specific tissue is "too short" for running, stretching in a valid method will improve it. In the screening section in Chapter 9, we'll put you through tests to see where you fall as a runner.

Tissue Stiffness—The Proper "Dose" of Stretching

How long should you hold a stretch? 10–20 seconds? Well—sorry, no. Research shows that significant improvements in tissue length occur when each muscle is lengthened for 3–5 minutes, 4–6 days a week. It takes sufficient time to shift the load on the tissue into the plastic range on the length-deformation curve (see Chapter 2 to refresh your memory).

How long until I begin to see improvements? Significant increases in length occur after 10–12 weeks of stretching. I know this is not what you wanted to hear, but it's the truth! Don't shoot the messenger. You can improve your soft tissue length, but it's not going to happen overnight. Let's make this simple: For shortened tissues, aim to hit three minutes of stretching almost daily, for ten weeks.

Is it best to stretch before or after my runs? Always stretch after your workout or race. Why? If you are about to draw a picture, the dumbest thing to do would be to whack your hand with a hammer twenty times, right? The swelling and pain in your hand would impair your fine motor control. Just the same, ripping (damaging) your muscles immediately prior to a workout doesn't really make sense does it? If the long-term goal is to increase soft tissue length, always do it after your run.

But I always feel better if I stretch before my run . . . you are telling me I should stop? Just as you warm up your car for a bit prior to gunning the gas pedal, your body needs to rev up as well. The body never works at 100 percent when cold. Stretching does not increase blood flow to the muscles; raising your heart rate does. A dynamic warm-up is a great way to wake up your nervous system. A dynamic warm-up is simply moving around, such as a light easy jog followed by some jumps or drills. If you like to do light or dynamic stretches to loosen you up prior to your workout, go for it.

What's so different about stretching "dynamically"? Dynamic stretches have a different purpose than long, sustained stretches. It would probably cut down on a great deal of confusion if these weren't called stretches at all. While stretching aims to improve tissue mobility, dynamic stretching aims to change the nervous system's *perception of tightness* in the muscle without actually causing any type of tearing and weakening of tissue structure. I wish they were called *dynamic trickery.* Think of rebooting your computer. This type of "stretching" helps awaken and reset the nervous system, and may actually improve neurologic control during your workout and run. They feature very short holds—from 1–15 seconds—and do not expose the tissue to enough of a load to shift its state on the load-deformation curve.

So what does dynamic or light stretching do then? When lengthening a tissue to end range, even for a short time, we have some effect on the neuromuscular system. If you remember our discussion on the Golgi tendon and muscle spindle in Chapter 3, you know that it is possible to alter their feedback and feed-forward activity with short stretches. Doing light stretches for 1–20 seconds, contract-relax stretches (when you contract a muscle briefly, it is always followed by a period of greater relaxation), reciprocal inhibition (where you try to contract the quad to get greater relaxation from the hamstrings; this is marketed as Active Isolated Stretching), and PNF (proprioceptive neuromuscular facilitation, which are specific diagonal movement patterns) are effective ways to trigger the nervous system.

Should I do this instead of static stretching? There is some resistance in the running community to the idea that static assessment of soft tissue length is not valid. Some coaches feel that runners move more when running than when performing the static test. Tissue length does *not* change during a run as compared with a static testing situation. Athletes who feel they are "stiff" respond well to dynamic techniques. In other words, their body feels as if it is tighter than it actually is. Running activates a number of reflexes and it inhibits this sensation of stiffness. This may actually enable the runner to move more while running than in their static assessment. Here's a good test to see if you could benefit from static stretching. When performing the tests in the screening section, try to contract the muscle for a second, and then relax. For example: When checking the hamstring length in Chapter 9, you'll lie on the ground and lift your leg up to seventy degrees. If you stop well short of this, try to firmly contract your hamstring for five seconds, relax, and then continue to raise the hamstring. If you notice a significant difference by doing this once or twice, it's obviously due to a change in perception of tightness and not a change in muscle length. Athletes that fall under this category feel that dynamic stretching in this manner loosens them up and gets them ready for a workout. These claims are valid based upon the change in neural tone.

So stiffness is bad? Actually, the contrary. Research shows that a stiffer muscle can better transfer elastic energy. Having a "stiffer" muscle that has full mobility is likely the optimal situation for runners. We'll discuss ways to increase stiffness in Chapter 6.

Why is having too much motion bad for me? Having more mobility than you need can actually create problems. If you talk to any physical therapist, you'll find that they treat almost as many injuries due to excessive mobility as they do to restriction of mobility. Movement without control is a recipe for disaster. Now if you are a runner and also happen to be a competitive gymnast then your personal mobility needs are greater. However, the increased mobility you have from gymnastics doesn't necessarily provide any tangible benefit to your running. To summarize tissue length, enough is critical, and more or less than this amount can be problematic.

- Having enough mobility to run introduces less compensatory motion through the musculoskeletal system, for a smoother forward progress.
- There is no research to show that more mobility than required for the running gait has any positive effect on performance or injury.
- Stretching is a valid way to improve specific limitations in soft tissue length when needed.
- If you feel pain or stiffness inside the joint while trying to stretch, it's likely a limitation in joint mobility. Contact your health care provider for help.
- Dynamic stretches, less than 20–30 seconds, cause short-term adaptations to improve neuromuscular function prior to a workout.
- Sustained holds of 3–5 minutes, 4–6 days a week for 10–12 weeks cause tissues to adapt by increasing length, and should be done following the run.

Tissue Glide—Why Soft Tissues Get Stuck and What We Can Do to Improve Them

Back when I was in school, I had this preconceived notion that a reduced flexibility in a body part was equal throughout the entire muscle and tendon. Basically, if the muscle or tendon was tight, then it was tight all the way through. Well, my newbie-mind was quite wrong. Even though you can bend down and touch your toes, it doesn't mean that the tension inside the hamstrings is uniform. As mentioned in chapters 2 and 3, scar tissue in random orientation sticks layers of the tissues together. This creates two problems:

1. Isolated areas of high stiffness are the first ones to become damaged. It's not good to keep all your stress in one place, right? Areas of the

muscle and tendon that are stuck down are stiff and under high loads, while other areas are under very little load. These areas of high stiffness can't adapt normally to the work/recovery cycles of training and can create injuries.

2. Stiff layers with less mobility can't perform at full capacity. You can't expect optimal performance out of damaged tissues.

So far, we've talked a lot about collagen's ability to move, and now we are going to dig a little bit deeper to see how this all plays out. And fixing these issues is one of the most powerful tools in your bag of tricks to optimize gains from training.

Time to wash the car. You turn on the hose and get a nice flow of H_2O pouring out. Since the inside diameter of the hose is the same throughout its length, there is equal pressure against the walls all the way through. *When collagen fibers are free to move and aligned in the same direction, equal load is distributed throughout.* So on you go, pulling, tugging, and twisting the hose so that you can reach all the sides of the car. Pretty much without fail, you'll pull and twist the hose in a certain way and the flow of water pressure will

Collagen Structure

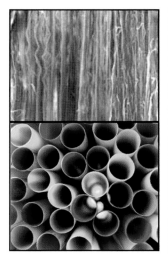
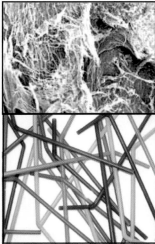

Healthy collagen, much like parallel straws, is aligned in a specific direction so it can respond to specific stresses. Damaged collagen fibers change their architecture and compromise tissue function. A random pattern of straws is weak and cannot tolerate much load.

drop considerably. The water is still on, but looking at the hose shows a kink somewhere along its length. *Sometimes the collagen healing process goes awry, and normal slide and glide is lost. Tissues become stuck together as extra bonds are formed between adjacent fibers that stiffen and limit their mobility.* The hose kink produces two major changes. First, the area around the kink is narrower. This means that pressure against the inside wall of the hose is much higher. Higher pressure for long periods of time can weaken the area and eventually cause it to rupture (tear). *Stiff tissue layers can't spread out the load as well, so some parts of the tissue inherit more strain than others. These higher strain zones are more prone to injury.* The second thing is that this narrowing produces less flow (output) from the hose. *Stiff layers with less mobility can't perform at peak capacity. You can't expect optimal performance out of damaged tissues.*

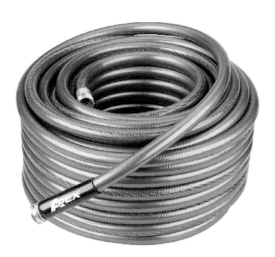

Will stretching free up these areas of high stiffness? Pull hard on a kinked hose. It actually makes the kink tighter. MRI imaging shows that stretching weakened and excessively stiff tissue produces weak and stiff tissue that is simply longer. The areas of high stiffness were never addressed and the chronic problem continues. You need to stop the wash job, find the kink, physically untwist it, and possibly even work it out if it's an old, worn-out hose. To improve tissue glide, find the specific spot of stiffness, and work it out. Once the random fibers have been broken up, uniform mobility is again present and the tissue is capable of peak performance.

Why did this excessive scar develop? I've always said that when you pop out of the womb at birth, they should ask you if you plan on being an endurance athlete. If your cry suggests yes, you should leave the hospital with a foam roller and a LAX ball as standard equipment. The training and recovery cycles of endurance athletes virtually guarantees soft tissue adhesions from excessive scarring. Training breaks the body down. Then it takes eleven to fourteen days for contractile proteins to repair the damage. I'm pretty sure that everyone reading this book works out more than once every week and a half. This means that subsequent training loads are applied before the body is ready for them, day after day, week after week, and year after year. Instead of specific repair in specific directions, the body throws in any attempt it can to keep things together during repair. Take all those straws we threw on the ground in Chapter 2 and spray adhesive all over them. Then throw more straws on top of them, and keep spraying on even more adhesive. Poor healing = poor mobility = parts can't do the job they were designed to do. After all, if you bind your buddy up in a straightjacket, he can't take a swing at you. Another friend has to set him free to let him do his thing . . . wait . . . seriously—you put your friend in a straightjacket? Maybe you deserve to get clocked!

Mobilizing the Scar: Seek and Destroy

Is there a best method to do this? Numerous groups have found trademark names to identify the proprietary tools and techniques they use. They claim to "improve fascial mobility" through the use of names like Active Release Therapy, Graston, ASTYM, and other techniques. I call my approach tissue flossing, but you can call it anything you want. No matter what the name, the premise is very simple and very similar: *free up tissue mobility where it's bound down*. While you can pay these folks $80 to $100 an hour to do this to you, you can do it yourself—it's free! In fact, I'd argue that periodic self-assessment of your body is critical and your responsibility as an athlete. If you can catch these issues while they are small, you can restore optimal tissue mechanics and function before they become a major issue. *Running is going to place lots of cumulative stress on the body*, and the body is going to scar to heal the area. However, the body can use some help to keep tissues supple and optimize its healing. Supple tissues work better.

Collagen Structure

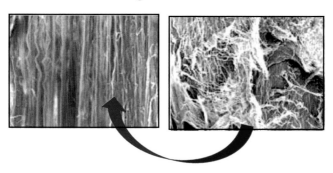

The goal of tissue mobilization is to get the collagen fibers to look and perform like they should. Fibers in parallel arrangement act uniformly.

While we will describe the process here, the best lesson you'll get is from feeling around and getting to know the stiff spots in your own body. Take your hand and lightly massage your forearm. Notice how the muscle bellies feel rather supple. Supple is good. Stiff is bad. It's pretty easy to self-diagnose excessively stiff tissues. Explore and poke around, trying to find any place in the lower body muscles that feel very sore or overly rigid.

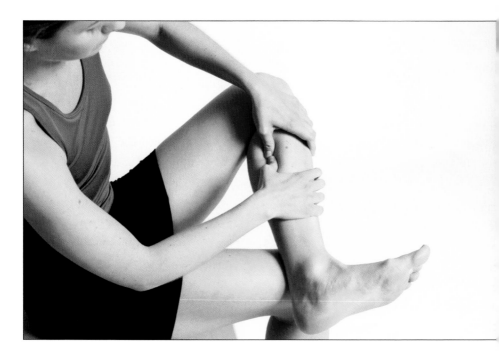

Self soft-tissue release of the posterior tibialis

Since shin splints are very common in runners, let's poke around the lower leg. While sitting, cross one leg over the other like you are reading the paper. Take your thumbs and press firmly on the inside of the shin (tibia).

Move up and down the ridge of the tibia feeling for quality and soreness as you go. Remember what supple tissue felt like in your forearm? If you find things that feel like climbing rope, or maybe a flank steak that was left on the grill for 24 hours, you have kinks. Simply compressing parts of the body shouldn't cause pain. In fact, some of you may roll your eyes back in your head doing this. That is *not OK* that areas of your body have gotten this stiff. It didn't hurt when you poked around your forearm, right? You want to mobilize the sticky layers until they become supple yet again. The only way to do it is to *do* it.

How do you do it? We'll go through this for numerous locations in the mobility assessment section, but for the shin it's pretty easy. It's really not rocket science and is amazingly successful. Take your thumbs and press into the stiff and sore areas. While maintaining firm pressure on the area, dorsiflex and plantarflex your ankle. This may feel quite sore at times, and that is OK. The combination of compression and active movement literally breaks up the stiff tissue. The rules are the same for any site. Position the joint so the tissue you want to work on is loose and relaxed. Apply firm pressure over the restriction and move the joint back and forth to shorten and lengthen it under your fingers and break it up.

Does tissue glide affect tissue length? Yes, indeed. If you free up the weak link in the chain, the whole chain can tolerate more load. So while stretching takes 10–12 weeks to improve tissue *length*, this scar mobilization technique improves in tissue *mobility* in a fraction of the time. I'm not always very patient, and I know you want quick results as well. By dedicating 3–5 minutes per area daily, you can expect to restore optimal tissue mobility in about 2–3 weeks.

OK, so tissue flossing helps correct chronic tightness, but should you wait until things are broken to pull it out of your bag of tricks? No! Many of you take your car in for periodic maintenance—doesn't your body demand the same level of respect to stay in tip-top shape? Ignoring routine checks on your car over time has a tendency to result in bigger, costly problems. A busted car requires you to take time out of your daily schedule to fix things, usually at a great cost. Don't wait until the body is injured to take it in for service. *Almost all endurance athletes will have excessive scar problems at various times.* Periodic checks of soft tissue mobility will identify small issues before they become bigger issues and cause injury. Stay ahead of the curve. The body is going to heal—that's a given. It's your responsibility to ensure that the tissues remain supple throughout the healing process. Optimal recovery of your tissues equals optimal performance so you can get more out of your training.

Tissue Mobility

- Tissue layers stuck together are compromised.
- The internal strain is not distributed evenly, forming focal areas likely to tear.
- Stuck tissues can't handle their normal demands and produce less output.
- Local restrictions in tissue mobility can limit tissue length.
- To reverse this process, the excess scar must be broken up manually.
- While stretching can improve gross tissue length with long holds over 10–12 weeks, the improvements in tissue mobility, and its net improvement on tissue length, can be obtained within weeks. Stop stretching, and start mobilizing!

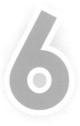

Dynamic Neuromuscular Strength—Make a Smarter, Stronger Spring

Flamingos are funny creatures, aren't they? Most of their body weight is in their torso, head, and wings, with two long impossibly slender legs supporting them. And they actually stand comfortably on one leg for long stretches of time—so much physical body mass, so eloquently balanced. To balance such a large weight on top of such a long narrow limb requires a certain amount of strength for sure, but more importantly, it requires control. Even if the flamingo could squat 400 pounds, it needs the precise

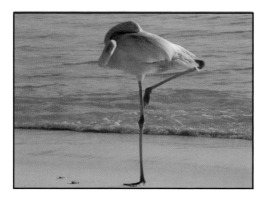

Despite their top-heavy body mass and long slender legs, this flamingo is stable. Runners, are you jealous?

control to make very minute adjustments in balance as the wind blows. Did you ever dream of flying like a bird? Well, let's just focus on standing like one first.

Phase 1: Poor Decisions in Muscle Control—Make Smarter Decisions

Michelle is a regionally competitive high school runner and cyclist. Lots of cycling and running volume mean she has gotten lots of strengthening of the muscles that move her forward. Due to this training, she is exceptionally fit, but is commonly plagued with injuries—especially right-sided patellofemoral pain—that force her to take time off.

One of the tests we'll present in the assessment section is the single-leg squat. The runner does a bunch of squats on one leg and watches for specific factors that show a lack of control in the stabilizing muscles. Michelle starts on her left leg. She is told to place her hands on her hips, stand on one leg, and complete eight squats. As she does this, we note that she does a good job keeping her torso and pelvis level. Her knee tracks so that it is above her foot and below the knee. Based on this criteria (we'll go over this test more in the intervention), we score her as a 6/6. Perfect. We then repeat this test on the right leg. Same instructions are given. This time, things look different. Michelle's torso leans a bit, her pelvis drops, and her knee dives to the inside. She scores a 3/6 on the right.

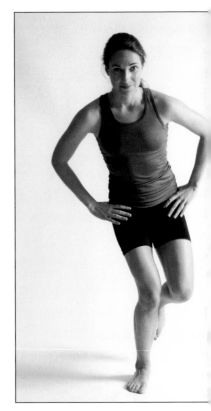

Next, we perform the bridge test. She moves up into bridge pose. We ask her what she feels, and she responds that her back is somewhat tight. We note that she has a big arch in her low back. We ask her to lift her right leg (so she is weight bearing on the left leg only) and despite the arched back, she does a good job of keeping her pelvis level for 30 seconds. We give Michelle a

Not a stable platform.

break and let her come back down. We then ask her to bridge up again, this time raising her left leg. As soon as she transfers her weight to the right leg and raises the left, we note that the pelvis rotates downward, and she reports a cramp in her right hamstring.

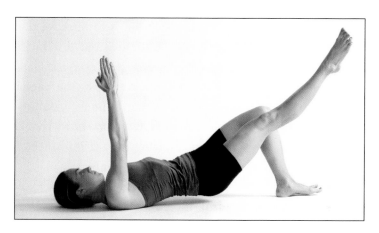

Breakdown in body position when simply raising one leg in bridge pose indicates pronounced deficits that will become magnified in gait.

Both tests show a consistent pattern. Michelle has deficient hip stability on the right ride. How does this play into the development of patellofemoral pain dysfunction? Ten years ago, you'd ask a clinician what to do about this, and they'd tell you to strengthen your quads. Is this really the right call? You have four muscles that make up the common muscle that we call the quadriceps. On the outside of the leg, you have a large muscle called the vastus lateralis and a much smaller muscle on the inside of the leg called the vastus medialis oblique. They would have told you that the large muscle on the outside is stronger than the muscle on the inside. This imbalance pulls the kneecap lateral and shifts the train (patella) lateral on the track (thigh). This explanation was accepted and sounded reasonable before the year 2000. If someone tells you this now, ask for another clinician. This person obviously hasn't read any literature on knee pain in the last ten years.

The past decade has shown the above explanation to be untrue. It is true that the lateral quad is much larger than the inner quad. But so what? The quads either contract as a whole or they don't. All four parts of the quad are innervated by the same nerve. While it's true that extensive swelling will shut off the inner quad slightly more than the lateral, you can't selectively isolate the different parts of the quad. So toss the above explanation out the window.

So what is the mechanism? As you run, the hips should rotate in and out as part of the normal shock absorption mechanics of the body. Research shows that runners with patellofemoral pain rotate more to the inside. This inward rotation of the hip shifts the groove in which the patella tracks. This shift in rotational alignment creates wear and tear on places the kneecap (the train) was not designed to be stressed. Therefore, the solution is to improve the function of hip muscles to stabilize the rotation and "straighten out the track." Thus the mantra becomes: *don't treat the train, treat the track.*

We are using this all-too-common pain in the front of the knee because research shows that it's the most common injury in runners, claiming over 20 percent of you as victims. And interestingly, research shows that this same movement pattern of pelvic drop and knee diving inward is also the mechanism of IT band problems, ACL tears, and medial shin splints.

In an ideal world, Michelle's hip muscles would control this excessive motion, eliminate the mechanism, and fix the problem. This requires an increase in coordination and recruitment of the hip stabilizer muscles. Michelle is a pretty smart girl. She talked to some folks and found some good exercises online. She did a bunch of side-lying leg lifts and a bunch of single-leg squats and a bunch of elastic band hip abduction exercises. So what happened? Well, after five weeks, she still had symptoms. In fact, things had gotten worse. She could still bike, but she had to stop running due to pain. She didn't understand. The tests she had done revealed weakness in her hip control, and she did specific things to improve it. She was confused.

I see a lot of people just like Michelle. They know what is going on and they are doing lots and lots of exercises to try to fix their limitations. A lot of people I see do great exercises, but they do them wrong. Poor practice equals poor execution. You see, Michelle has F.A.T.S. I didn't say she *is* fat; I said she *has* F.A.T.S., or Female Adolescent Texting Syndrome.

OK—so I made up the name for this "diagnosis" myself, but problems with postural control run deep, really deep, and can ruin your chances of getting over chronic injury. F.A.T.S. is a friendly way to discuss a common presentation that was coined decades ago as Lower Quarter Crossed Syndrome. This is the second biggest problem I see in runners. Number one is a lack of hip extension but since number one basically creates number two, they are pretty related.

What does good postural control look like? Take out a copy of *National Geographic*. Somewhere in there you'll find a picture of a woman in Africa walking out in the fields with absolutely perfect posture, likely balancing between 30–40 pounds of flour or grain on her head on her way back to the

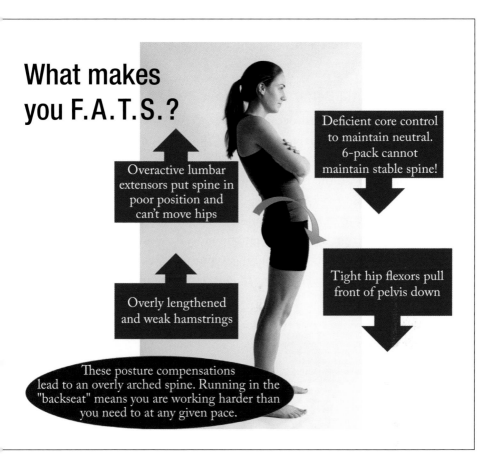

What makes you F.A.T.S.?

Overactive lumbar extensors put spine in poor position and can't move hips

Deficient core control to maintain neutral. 6-pack cannot maintain stable spine!

Overly lengthened and weak hamstrings

Tight hip flexors pull front of pelvis down

These posture compensations lead to an overly arched spine. Running in the "backseat" means you are working harder than you need to at any given pace.

village. Living in a society like this keeps you "active." You don't sit all day in a car commuting, at a desk in school, or playing Xbox because your life is quite different. And you've figured out that to carry a huge load on your head, you need to align your posture in neutral so that the load comes through the spine. If you keep your alignment "stacked," it takes less muscle control to carry the rice a mile back to your village.

Contrast this with our typical young high school girl. She stands knees locked, pelvis tilted forward, and rounded, slumped shoulders. And then mom says, "Don't slouch Michelle. Get your shoulders back!" So Michelle arches her back to get her shoulders back . . . at the expense of compromising her spine position. Michelle texts like this, stands like this, walks like this. This posture, right or wrong, feels like home. Posture is not static, it's dynamic. The body makes thousands of tiny contractions every second to keep your position in check. If these contractions occur in a faulty position, you reinforce faulty position with your muscle memory. And some tissues get tight and some get overly lengthened. Any guess on what kind of posture Michelle is going to run with? She's going to stick with what she "knows." So why should we teach her something different?

Core Control—Put a Better Brain in Your Bucket

The buzzword of the last decade has been *core*; core strength, core stability. Thousands of "core exercises" out there and thousands of products on nightly infomercials are designed to improve our core. Before you spend three EZ-payments of $19.99 on the next video or device, we should likely review what core control really is.

There are many muscles in the midsection. All muscles do is shorten. When they shorten, one end of the muscle moves towards the other. Some of these muscles like your rectus abdominus (your six-pack), your internal and external obliques, and your erector spinae muscles cause us to move. For example,

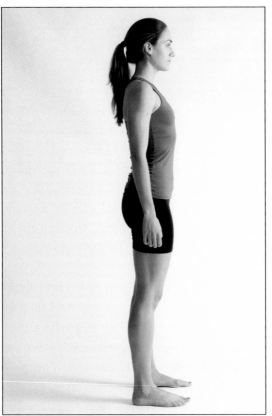
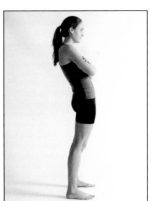
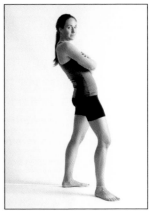

The position we stand in all day is our baseline. Which position do you think is better for our bodies?

hen you contract your six-pack, you either flex your torso forward towards the elivs, or tuck your pelvis underneath to flatten the low back. In either case, ie rectus abdominus contraction produced a distinct movement—a change in osition. The problem is that the rectus abdominus and your obliques are more ıst twitch, not postural muscles. By definition, you cannot depend on them to old your posture in line all day or during a run. They will fatigue and your osition and economy will change.

Other muscles in the midsection don't really have much of an effect on hanging position of your upper body or lower body. The transversus abdomi-ıus, the multifidi, and the pelvic floor are more concerned with keeping things ı position. The multifidi are thin muscles in the back of your spine. They have ie greatest proprioceptive nerves of any muscle in the body. They monitor ie position of each and every vertebrae in the spine. As you move, they tell our brain exactly how much each vertebrae moved on another vertebrae. Some f this information goes to our brain, and some of it goes into reflexes. Your ·ansversus has a different job. It runs around the body similarly to the way a orset wraps around the body. If you tighten the corset on a woman's dress, it revents movement. When the transversus fires, it doesn't change the position f the body either. The true definition of core control is how well you can keep our upper body stable on the lower body.

OK—time for an example to pull this together. Look at a toy plastic bucket. he cylinder formation of the bucket gives it strength. If you place your hands round the bucket and push uniformly around the entire cylinder of the wall ou'll be amazed at how much force you can push with. When you evenly dis-ibute forces around a structure, it can withstand a lot of load prior to failure. his is why the spine works well when in neutral. Neutral is slightly different for ach and every one of us, and that's OK.

Next, take a finger and poke at the side of the bucket until it gives. You'll otice that the bucket partially collapses on itself. The sides of the bucket are ow actually weaker. This is similar to bending the spine in any given direction. Vhen you've moved out of your neutral spine position, you have weakened the :ability of the core.

Core control has nothing to do with how many crunches, twists, or super-ıans you do on a daily basis. In fact, overstrengthening the spinal "movers" ·ith weak stabilizers actually creates large problems in core control. Remember, ıe "movers" will fatigue as they are not postural muscles. Yes, even if you do 00 crunches a day. Ripped abs do not equal good core control. Why not?

The key feature of core control is not strength, but timing. Research show that good core control is actually a *feed-forward* response. If I move my arm out to the side, my brain knows that moving the limb away from my center of mass will change my balance point, and it will naturally kick on my true core stabilizers 40 milliseconds prior to me moving my arm. In the lower body, 110 milliseconds before I move my leg, my brain kicks on to keep my body stable and in line. Proper stabilization depends on proactive, not reactive control. There is some pretty complex coordination going on here, and your transversus and multifidi actually have their own independent nervous system pathways to sort things out.

People with posture dysfunction (F.A.T.S.) and back pain lasting longer than four weeks don't follow the rules. Their coordinated control of the spinal stabilizers becomes *inhibited* (or disconnected). These people *do* have core muscles, and they *do* contract just as forcefully as people with normal core stability. However, we see a *shift in timing*. Instead of firing ahead of the movement, the muscles fire *too late*. What does this mean? The take-home message here is that core control is about proximal stability prior to distal mobility. All the muscles in the lower extremity attach directly or indirectly to the pelvis. If the coordination of the core is off, your house is not built on a solid slab, but wobbly, dry-rotting piers.

Let's go back to Michelle. She had problems with lateral and rotational hip control, and worked the muscles that fire around the hip. There is a problem with this approach, though. Muscles don't work in isolation. They work together in a precisely controlled manner. If she cannot achieve proper posture and core control, her spine and pelvis are always unstable, meaning that the muscles that control the hip are also unstable. She can't isolate the *proper* stabilizing muscles to keep things in check and finds a way to cheat. And cheaters never win.

Michelle finds a recommended physical therapist in her area. This PT points out that she needs to work from the "inside out." By working on controlling her core stability first, the hip muscles have a better base from which to operate. Since stance times are so short in running, proper stabilization needs to occur *before you contact the ground*. If there is no free-forward control, you'll never be able to correct your mechanics during the stance phase. Timing is everything.

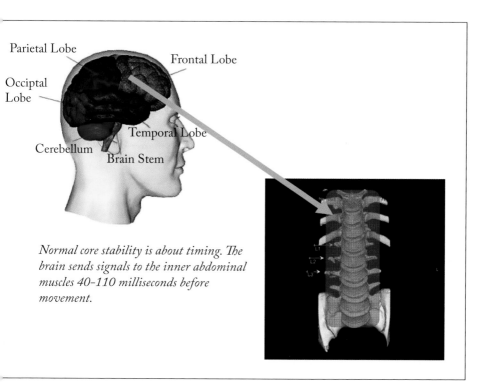

Parietal Lobe

Frontal Lobe

Occiptal
Lobe

Temporal Lobe

Cerebellum

Brain Stem

Normal core stability is about timing. The brain sends signals to the inner abdominal muscles 40-110 milliseconds before movement.

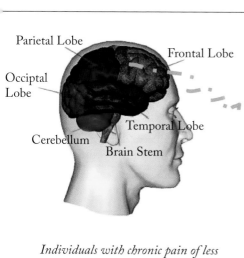

Parietal Lobe

Frontal Lobe

Occiptal
Lobe

Temporal Lobe

Cerebellum

Brain Stem

Individuals with chronic pain of less than 2–4 weeks or excessive posture dysfunction lose feed-forward muscle control. The core muscles do fire, but they fire too late to stabilize the spine

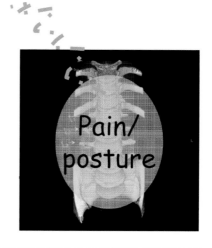

Pain/
posture

Turning on Your Core Muscles

Practicing proper core muscle activation is usually a very telling process. Athletes with good core function have absolutely no problem isolating the deep abdominal muscle called the transversus. On the flip side, it can be very challenging for athletes with chronic inhibition from poor posture or back pain to identify them. Proper training must be tailored to each individual. Here's the easiest way to try to get you to isolate your inner abdominal muscle.

Sit up straight or stand. Place each index finger on the prominent bump in front of the pelvis (near the beltline). Then slide them straight up, about one inch. This is the best location to feel the transversus without feeling too much of the obliques. Now make a face like you are about to say cheese for the camera. Your lips will pucker outward like you are blowing on a horn. We actually don't want to do this because you'll use the wrong muscles. So keep your teeth together, but let your lips relax. Next place your tongue up against the front of your teeth so it almost blocks the air from leaving your mouth. OK—now you are set up take a regular inhalation and then a long slow exhalation. As you exhale, press your tongue against the front of your mouth. With the tongue providing pressure, the transversus has some pressure to push back against. If you are doing everything correctly, you should be able to feel the muscles poking outward into your fingers. While this breathing trick is the way to find your transverus, aim to tighten it at will. You should be able to uncouple your muscle control from your breathing. Activating this muscle is like kindergarten: you should never go to first grade without learning essential skills. Skilled control of the transversus is a part of each and every exercise in this book and something you should be able to do when running.

Changing Neuromuscular Control: Making Muscles Smarter

We know that running demands we generate large forces. And we need to make smarter decisions in our *neuromuscular* control to avoid instability. Muscular control is your first and best line of defense. However, we often forget that muscles only turn on and off in very precise amounts when told to by the nervous system. The nervous system allows you to adjust your force. It's the reason you can catch an egg without crushing it. You don't go from completely relaxed to full contraction each and every time you move, so the brain's ability to coordinate and stabilize the muscular force results in a state of *dynamic stability*. Correct the imbalance, and correct your chances of developing a host of injuries.

What changes in these neuromuscular training programs?

The cornerstone of dynamic strength revolves around the ability to make rapid microcorrections to keep joints properly aligned. You shouldn't need someone to tell you if you are in good position or not; you should be able to *sense* it internally. Our body comes prewired to do just that. If you do need someone to help you find the correct spine, hip, or foot position, no problem—it's just evidence that you have improvement coming your way after you set aside some time to work on it. We determine our joint position and overall body orientation by combining information from three primary sources:

1. **Vestibular System** (inner ear)—If you are standing still, inner ear fluid is still. If you turn your head suddenly, the inner ear fluid swirls. This information goes to your brain to help determine acceleration and change in position.
2. **Visual**—We use our eyes to orient our head and trunk and let us know which way is "up."
3. **Somatosensory**—You "feel" the ground. You have sensory receptors in your skin that allow you to feel joint position, light and deep pressure, vibration, heat, cold, etc. This sensation goes a long way to improve your tactile feedback to help you remain stable.

These pathways talk to each other and are even modified slightly by things like head position and pressure to determine body position. If these three systems "agree," we get clear signals to control the body in stance. If they reveal differences, then the brain gets confused. If you are on a merry-go-round, your eyes see you are spinning, your somatosensory system feels the body turning, and your vestibular system says you are spinning. Everything is fine. If you stop, your eyes and somatosensory system say you have stopped, but your inner ear fluid is still swirling—signals don't agree . . . and you become dizzy.

So why is it harder to close your eyes in single-leg balance? Most folks are visually dominant. They rely highly on their eyes to find their position in space. The problem with this is that it's "slow." You need to see information, process it in the visual part of your brain, then send a signal to the part of your brain that controls motion (motor cortex) to make a correction. Somatosensory nerves are hardwired to transfer information through the body faster than any other nerve type. There is a direct relay between the sensory and motor reflexes both inside and outside the brain. Fast info in equals fast info out. This results in rapid "microcorrections" of position. Let's use an example.

If you look at skiers, surfers, skateboarders, white water paddlers—they all have something in common—they need to make positional corrections *very* quickly—faster than they can see and adjust. They get good feedback about the position of their body from their hard ski edge (transferred up through a very stiff plastic boot) or the rail of the surfboard (transferred through their bare feet). Each and every time they practice their sport they are refining their position sense by "feeling" where the body is. They consistently train and improve their somatosensory system.

A Higher Level of Thinking for Exceptional Athletes—How'd They Get There?

Have you ever seen Cirque du Soleil? It's an amazing group of true athletes. Not only can they do headstands, they can do headstands on top of someone else riding a unicycle. Not only can they blast twenty feet into the air on that floppy bamboo pole, but they can land delicately on a pole or some other ridiculously small object or another person. Their movements are the textbook definitions of coordination, timing, and skill. The slightest error in the landing mechanics is enough to change all of that in a split second. How do these people learn their skills? Not by throwing 300 pounds on their back and pounding out squats. They've improved their coordination through practice in different situations. Sure, specific practice is important. If your job is to bound off the bamboo pole, do a double flip, and land perfectly in someone else's outstretched hand, well, you better practice this unique skill. *Good* athletes practice specific skills. *Great* ones practice many skills.

Let's say that last season, you were the woman who was spinning inverted on the rings. You'll tap into your sense of body awareness and visual sighting skills that you gained when working on the rings and take this with you to your next stunt. Highly skilled athletes don't view situations in isolation. By exposing themselves *often* to *many different conditions*, they have a very refined muscle memory. Highly skilled athletes don't think "*how* am I going to do this right?" They just *do* it right. The skill goes from the conscious to the unconscious. The more different stuff you do, the better control you have of your parts in all situations. Controlled parts can transfer and produce extraordinarily high forces with minimal strain on the body.

So what does this mean for you? To do a *great* job controlling your body when running and avoiding form changes with fatigue requires you to invest some time. At first, practicing new skills is hard and may be actually less efficient. Because of the increased cognition or thought that learning new skills requires, the athlete may in fact be less efficient at their particular sport because they are "thinking" so much about the way in which they move. If you introduce the subject of posture correction to your milers one morning, don't expect them to be able to perfectly carry this over into their speedwork session that same day. They'll need to practice this by just walking and sitting before they can achieve it at race intensity. Depending on speed, stance phases during running are between 0.12-0.25 seconds. Even at the slower end, this is quicker than most of you (well, myself anyway) can think. In the 0.17 seconds when you complete a stance phase, you don't have time to contact the ground and then say, "OK, self—straighten trunk, activate glute, drive big toe down, and . . ." You get the point. Things just need to happen in the right sequence and in the right amounts.

Correcting imbalances is all about moving *smarter*, not *stronger*. You should never attempt high intensity strength and plyometric exercises until you have mastered specific stabilization of the parts. Why? *Unstable levers cannot tolerate high loads.* If you can't generate *specific force from the right muscles* to stabilize against these loads, the body compensates. Athletes develop poor movement skills because they don't know any better. Simply adding *more volume, more intensity, and more challenge to runners with poor local control is about as effective as drunk driving*. Things will go catastrophically downhill at some point. Athletes should only progress to true strengthening activities when they know they are moving correctly. In Chapter 9, we'll discuss specific ways to identify what your individual limiters are and specific ways to improve them.

Women are at a higher risk of developing a host of lower leg injuries compared with men. This high risk is not really due to inferior parts, but rather inferior control of their parts. All the research shows that women have different muscle firing strategies than men. In general, women allow their leg to rotate and dive inwards. This is the exact movement pattern that *causes* ACL tears, patellofemoral pain syndrome, shin splints, and ITB problems.

What if you did something on a daily basis that actually made you move wrong? Anyone wear skirts? Sorry ladies, I know they look cute, but skirts are creating movement problems that you aren't aware of. Skirts force you to keep your legs superclose together with your knees crashing inward. This pattern has become part of your muscle memory as you've gotten used to sitting, standing, and walking this way. This muscle memory transfers into running as well.

Looking pretty in skirts is great, but when you switch that skirt for your running shorts, you've got to release your inner Lara Croft and get down to business. I'm not going to ask you to fight fashion, but I also don't want you to fight your body. Practice proper squat technique to make those muscles *smarter*. Knowing where your body *should be* will reverse these movement habits and decrease your chance of injury.

Muscle Memory Training: Progress

Learning to move smarter, just like any topic in school, requires you to start with the basics and move upward and onward from there. While everyone wants to be the guy in the gym doing squats on the Swiss ball, the only thing you'll get good at is falling on your head. Let's say you were like Michelle and had a poor score on the single-leg squat test. Doing more squats with your knee crashing to the inside is only going to reinforce the idea that it's OK to squat with your knee crashing into the inside.

Break the task down to the lowest level you can complete *successfully*. People learn best from positive feedback, not getting yelled at for screwing up. It is best done with a high volume of tasks that you *can* accomplish successfully, rather than try and fail at something too hard; focus on your limiters and build up.

If you are working on single-leg balance, start with just balancing. Not your "I'm-rocking-back-and-forth-like-a-weeble-wobble" reactive balance, but your "proactive balance." Proactive balance means: "I know what to do to keep my body stable—I can microcorrect to improve my stability." Start by working on quiet stance first. Think about spreading your toes out wide to maximize the width of your foot. Try to push your big toe down—not curling, just down as you keep it straight (we'll cover exactly how to do this in the testing section). Increasing the muscle control inside the foot makes you hyperaware of your position sense. You need to get a feel for this skill often to keep building up that mental database of tricks. Research shows it takes *4,000-6,000 reps* to change muscle memory. Do lots of volume in small doses to prevent the brain from getting fatigued. Instead of trying to balance on one leg for ten minutes each night, it's better to do it twenty times a day for 30 seconds.

As quiet stance improves, motor learning research tells us to make things more complex. Try closing your eyes, adding rotation, throwing a ball with a partner or against the wall, or try to slightly pronate and supinate the foot to help find the neutral position of the joint. Add firm unstable surfaces like rocker boards and upside-down BOSUs. Add jumping and jumping with rotation. The more varied the training opportunity, the more strategies you'll have in your mental database to improve control.

Getting in tune with your somatosesory system will reduce your visual dependency and improve your perception of *feel*. Because in the end, it's not *telling* you what to do that improves your balance and proprioception. The more skilled an athlete is, the more we need to shut our mouths and simply enable the athlete to find their correct position and build their own muscle memory around that perception. Refined motor skills are like "autopilot." Even in light of fatigue, you'll know how to correct your form. Think about some of the best performances you've ever done. What were you thinking about? Most successful athletes can't even remember what they were focusing on. They were in "the zone" and just let their bodies perform using the skills they learned through practice.

No this isn't "cross-training" —it's *complementary training*. Running is a pretty constrained movement pattern that tends to ignore our comprehensive athletic skill development. We need to expand your skill set. Go outside your comfort zone and push the limits of your stabilizing muscles. It pays off in spades. Research shows *excellent* results in neuromuscular training programs. What do I mean by excellent results? How about decreased injury rates, improvement in speed, agility, vertical jump, and contact times: elements of skill that will benefit runners of all levels.

○———————○

Can't I Just Go Straight To the Gym and Hit the Machines?

Machine weights have gained a large following due to the misconception that there is less chance for injury. Lifting weights on the machine allows the runner to push as hard as he or she can while being completely free of stabilizing the weight. Remember a quote we've come back to often: High forces through unstable levers are a recipe for disaster. The constrained movement on machine weights completely ignores the control and movement skill aspect of lifting weights. While increasing the true strength of a muscle is good, it's refining of movement skills that produces a more well-rounded athlete, one that can respond instantly to a stumble on the pavement, uneven terrain, or the effects of fatigue during a race. So what does this mean? Skip the machines. You'll get better carry-over of your strengthening program while controlling your body in stable and unstable situations than from simply moving the weight stack up and down.

Optimizing Energy Transfer: Hold the Human Slingshot Steady

So far our discussion on dynamic stability has focused on injury reduction. We haven't mentioned that improving control and coordination of our stabilizing muscles also impacts performance. Yes, that's right. All of this balance and stability training will actually improve your PR.

One of the main ways in which we run is by using elastic energy. We are going to elaborate on this a lot more when we get to the gait chapter (Chapter 8), but for now, let's look at a simple scenario. Go into your attic and find the slingshot you had as a kid, and grab a rock. Then go outside so you don't break a vase or a mirror in your house.

To launch the slingshot, you must first stabilize the end with one hand. The more you pull back the elastic end of the slingshot, the more elastic energy you store. If your lead hand stabilizes the slingshot, all this force is transferred to the rock upon release. *Whap!* —you'll likely hit your tree. When the stabilizing muscles in the body (base of slingshot) provide proximal stability, it results in optimal transfer of stored elastic energy from the tendon (elastic band) to move the body. However, if you can't generate enough stability and strength to control the handle, you can't stabilize the transfer of energy. The band flops around as it is released and doesn't release as much energy to the rock. Moving the body forward requires some type of force. If you can't take advantage of the elastic energy, you must generate more force from your muscles, and this costs more metabolic energy. Improving muscular stability of the limbs improves elastic energy transfer within the runner.

Main Points:

- Dynamic stability defines how well a runner stabilizes the body as they move it forward.

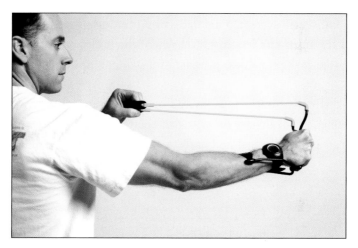

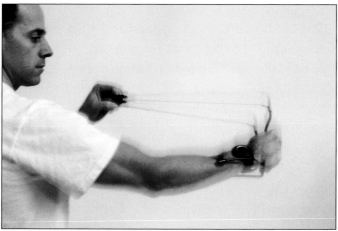

If the muscles "hold it steady," you get better energy transfer from the slingshot.

- Repetitive forces of running applied through unstable levers are a mechanism for disaster. Joint stability requires active neuromuscular control.
- The large imbalance between muscles that move the runner forward and muscles that stabilize the parts of the body is one of the biggest causes of injuries in the running athlete.
- A failure to achieve a stable chassis results in high forces transferring through unstable levers—a recipe for disaster. This results in overloaded tissues and poor energy transfer through muscles and tendons.
- Efficient neuromuscular control improves performance by effectively transferring elastic loads between the musculotendonous tissues; this minimizes internal work by the body.
- Improvements in this active stabilization come from refinements in the neuromuscular system. This occurs by training proprioception.
- Find the most challenging level where the athlete *can* accomplish the proposed task and work on increasing volume to build the mental database.
- The difficulty and/or load should only be advanced when the new movement skill has become part of the muscle memory, which the runner can internally feel and correct on their own.

Training Toys

I get asked by a lot of high school coaches, "What are the best core exercises for my team?" I tell them all the same thing: "Buy a bunch of longboard skateboards, stand-up paddle boards, indo-boards, and Swiss balls." The coach laughs and says, "OK, uh . . . thanks," and thinks I'm joking. They always say, "But I don't want the kids to get hurt!" Well, I don't either; that's why we are having this conversation! It's easier for kids to tap into their movement skills because they likely were on a skateboard a year or two ago. It's a bit "fresher" in their heads.

High school kids as a whole aren't that motivated to do an exercise; they want to do some type of game or skill. They actually really enjoy playing on this type of stuff. Next practice give the team a choice: A)

Everyone on the team has to balance on the Swiss ball on hands and knees and "walk" the ball down to the other side of the field, or B) Eight reps of 30-second planks. They'll get a better core workout doing the Swiss ball race, and I can almost guarantee you that they'll find a Swiss ball and practice between now and the next workout. When was the last time the whole team was motivated enough to do extra planks on their own? Make it fun and kids will stick with it. And if more of this was done now, we'd see runners heading on to college with better balance, proprioception, and lateral and rotational plane stability to better prepare them for the higher F.I.T. expected of them. And what kid doesn't want to rally around slalom cones on the skateboard as part of their warm-up?

Phase 2: Intense Strength in the Running Athlete — Increasing the Size of Your Spring

So you've practiced some single-leg balance control. You've practiced proper squat form (more on this in the intervention section). You can sense internally when you are doing it right and when you are defaulting back to your old habits. No athlete should advance to higher level resistance training until they can sense correct versus incorrect movement for themselves. Defaulting back to your old rusty self after you slap some weight on your shoulders brings you right back to the starting point. Yes, correcting movement skills takes some time. However, when you *are* ready . . . look out! You'll find that your performance ceiling with proper technique is significantly higher than your current ceiling.

The very definition of strength is the force produced per cross-sectional area. Bigger muscles produce bigger force. Pretty simple, right? At the start of this chapter we identified the exact loads that the body must stabilize against. Wouldn't increasing maximal strength help all runners? Or let's go ahead and introduce the point that the majority of old school coaching lore revolves around. If there is no correlation between 10K times and heavy lifting, why should runners lift weights? Close your eyes—right now you can see your old high school coach smirking at you, can't you? He says, "Runners run—all that lifting stuff doesn't translate to running." Well, I'm happy to report that the last decade has given us some very interesting data to support the idea that resistance training not only increases a runner's strength, but it also improves running economy. If some of you are against weight training that's fine, but I guess that means you are against performing at your peak potential as well.

In most sports, absolute force production is not the key factor. Rather, the ability to generate this force *quickly* is more critical. The definition of power is force generated over a given time. Imagine having a bigger spring.

Running faster requires the ability to produce greater force in the vertical, braking, and acceleration directions. Every single runner in the world, irrespective of style, increases these values when going faster and decreases them when running slower. The quest for improved performance requires more and better coordinated recruitment of the runner's muscle mass. So how does a runner maximize his muscle fiber recruitment?

1. **Run fast**—Since running faster requires more strength and thus more fiber to be recruited, you should just run fast all the time, right? While running fast demands more muscle mass, it also introduces *taxing physiologic stress* that cannot be sustained daily. Speedwork done in the right dose, and the right time, is the best way to optimize your muscle fiber recruitment while running.

2. **Run hills**—Raising the body's center of mass up the hill increases the force the runner must produce, thus increasing muscle fiber utilization. Hills are a great way to increase the force demand of running while running, but again, at the expense of *greater physiologic fatigue*.

3. **Weights**—Weight training (at high intensity) requires the runner to produce forces well above those seen during running. It's possible to activate a *very* high percentage of the runner's muscle mass, with *minimal physiologic fatigue*. When applied in the correct F.I.T., it's a great training tool to better develop the runner.

The sets and reps of your weight training affect the mechanical and neural stress placed on the body. The majority of runners aim for high reps and low weight. I'm going to chalk this strategy up to a combination of ignorance, "safety" (fear of going heavy and straining a muscle), and the magazines telling you to do it. Let's explore the science behind sets, reps, and weight.

The low-weight/high-repetition training that most runners adopt is targeted towards muscular endurance. It places about the same mechanical stress or even less!) on the body that we see during running. Since it's best to have ports-specific training, running is likely a better method to improve muscular ndurance. The literature has less support for low-weight/high-repetition train- ng as an effective way to significantly improve the force and speed generation f the muscles. While high-rep, no-weight training is the preferred way to lay foundation of improved *coordination and movement skills*, this one-sided ap- roach doesn't fully develop the body. If the goal is to improve performance by apidly activating and recruiting more muscle mass, *there really is no place for ow-weight, high-repetition training.*

Does this mean we should always advocate heavy lifting? No. As mentioned t length in the first half of this chapter, the first step is moving *smart*. Run- ers in general have a lot of bad habits and movement skills that need to be cleaned up" before any higher intensity type program is begun. If the goal is o improve *muscle coordination and movement skills*, then no-weight, high-rep raining is the appropriate method to allow the athlete numerous chances to eel their form and alter their neuromuscular recruitment. The tests in this ook can highlight what your individual neuromuscular needs are as they relate o running. Once the "skill" of the movement or exercise is learned, it's time to rogress.

Optimal Sets and Reps for Specific Resistance Training Goals

Goal	Sets	Reps
Improve Power	3–6	2–5, as fast as possible
Improve Strength	2–4	5–8, speed less of an issue
Improve Muscular Endurance	1–3	12–28, done slowly

Gains in true strength come from placing a stress on the body that is so reat, it causes it to increase the fiber size. This is called *hypertrophy*. This ncrease in size comes with an improved ability to generate force. If the goal is ctivation of almost all the muscle mass, lifting heavy weights is the key (with orrect form).

Hypertrophy is important for two reasons:

1. Ever heard the riddle: "What puts more force per square area, a woman in stilettos or an elephant?" While the elephant of course weighs more,

the four very large feet provide a large area to spread out the load. Contrast this with even a relatively lightweight collegiate distance runner going out for a night on the town, and you'll see that less weight spread through a tiny contact point is actually more force per area. A given amount of running F.I.T. on small muscles and tendons results in high forces inside the tissue. The larger cross-sectional area of muscle that develops as a result of resistance training yields less peak tissue strain for the same running F.I.T. A positive adaptation of strength training is that hypertrophy helps spread out forces more and results in less tissue damage.

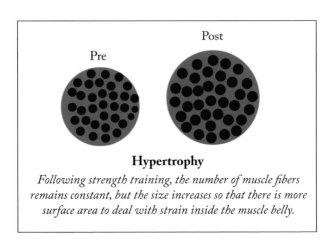

Hypertrophy

Following strength training, the number of muscle fibers remains constant, but the size increases so that there is more surface area to deal with strain inside the muscle belly.

2. Research shows that we lose strength and lean body mass at a rate much faster than any of you would like to know . . . even if you keep running. Mile after mile, running isn't really enough of a stimulus to strengthen the body. Some type of lifting program becomes more and more critical as the age of the runner increases. Research has shown that even men in their eighties can develop muscle mass through resistance training. Adding lean muscle mass burns more calories at rest, which helps combat the natural slowing of our metabolism as we age. It's no fountain of youth, but it can minimize your losses.

Should Kids Lift Weights?

When I was younger, I was told something that a lot of you may have heard as well: Lifting weights stunts your growth. Not only is this untrue, it's actually 180 degrees backwards. The American College of Sports Medicine has an official position paper on resistance training for kids. Lifting weights actually increases hormones related to bone mineral density, and increasing lean body mass (muscle mass) further increases signals to increase bone mineral density. Further, their bodies are changing rapidly; varied activities such as weight-lifting will improve their coordination and movement skills during these fast growth years. When taught properly, weight training is a safe training method with long-term benefits for kids.

Phase 3: Boing!—Getting a Faster *Spring* Out of Your Spring

Despite the need for increased force from muscles to run fast, peak strength is not, and should not be, the sole emphasis of a runner's weight training. Sport performance does not typically depend on the maximum amount of strength that the athlete can produce, but rather the power. Power is the force applied over a specific time. Running at 7.2 mph, the runner is only in contact with the ground for about 0.17 seconds. This is a pretty short time. The quicker and more coordinated the athlete can produce their force during this short contact period, the better the control during the activity. To maximize power, the emphasis is on moving the weight quickly (while maintaining control of the weight).

Plyometrics require rapid generation of force and improve power transfer through the body. Try asking a group of distance runners to jump for max vertical height. You'll rarely be impressed. The inability of most runners to generate vertical force for liftoff is rather perplexing since running is a just a bunch of single-leg hops. While peak vertical height should not be the end goal for runners, rapid delivery of muscular energy is. Improving the runner's ability to deliver explosive energy makes a difference from the 100-meter sprint all the way through the ultra distance.

Training for power requires very little time. While the intensity should be near explosive speeds, the minimum effective dose for power training is quite low. The only problem we see with plyometrics is that runners aren't ready for them. The stronger spring can't release its force rapidly unless it has a stable foundation. Complimentary skills make a well-rounded athlete. Train 'em. Do more different stuff.

This chapter has still not answered a question it proposed earlier: The research has shown that running economy improves following high intensity resistance training (and plyometrics too), but how? Does it improve your VO2? No, it does not. Will it impact your lactate threshold? There is evidence that it will if the runner is relatively untrained to begin with, but it's not overwhelming. So then what is left?

In Chapter 2, we introduced the idea that specific resistance training for strength and power can, in fact, improve the runner's ability to recruit muscle mass for improved force generation. However, don't think that the neuromuscular stage is over and you can move on to a new topic. High-intensity strength training and plyometrics demand a higher percentage of fibers to contract at once. Performing these high-intensity lifts further refines the neuromuscular control. This high-intensity lifting for speed *fine-tunes* our muscular stiffness so that we can produce full force very rapidly. In fact, training in this fashion allows runners to adopt faster stance times without a decrease in efficiency (contrary to commonly held beliefs, very short stance times are actually *less* efficient unless specific aims are taken to optimize recoil).

Remember the energy transfer discussion we had? Stiffer limbs do a better job of transferring force through the tendon and require less force to be internally generated by the muscle (which costs energy). Further, the ability to recruit large volumes of muscle mass provides a strength reserve that can help minimize the effects of fatigue and leave something in the tank for a sprint finish. So although hypertrophy is a positive adaptation of resistance training, it's not the one *most* critical to runners.

Visualizing Your Training

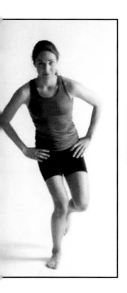

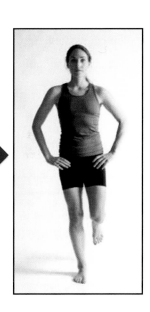

Making muscles smarter improves the foundation

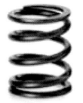

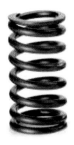

Improving strength and speed improves stiffness

It's simple math!

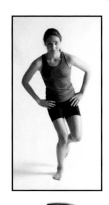

Unstable dynamic
control

Stable dynamic
control

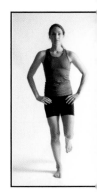

Small spring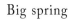

+

- Inefficiency and weakness
- High chance of injury

Small spring

+

- Less injury risk
- Poor performance

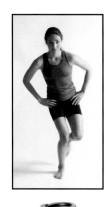

Unstable dynamic
control

Stable dynamic
control

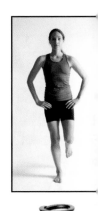

Big spring

+

- High forces through unstable levers
- High injury risk

Big spring

+

- Minimal injury risk
- Maximum performance

Smarter, Stronger Springs

The best athletes in the world constantly refine their technique and skills. High-level resistance training is a valid way to *tune* your elasticity and *refine* your motor skills.

The Strengthening Solution

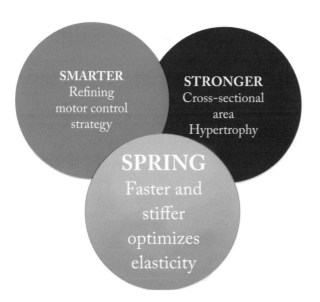

SMARTER
Refining
motor control
strategy

STRONGER
Cross-sectional
area
Hypertrophy

SPRING
Faster and
stiffer
optimizes
elasticity

We began by discussing that motion of the neuromuscular system is not "on" or "off." It's refined over the years by practicing lots of different skills. The more varied your training, the better muscle memory you'll develop. High forces through unstable parts will cause breakdown. Improved control not only minimizes the chance of injury, it also helps transfer elastic energy throughout the body when running. You don't get the V8 engine until you've learned how to control V8 power. When the runner has reached the point of autopilot, they are ready to include high-intensity resistance training programs in their routine.

Differences Between Men and Women

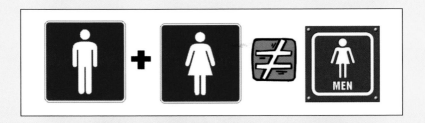

Every issue of every magazine has products "specifically for the unique needs of a woman!" Yes, these marketing folks are *very* good at attracting attention from the softer sex. One company claims that their shoes target "the unique needs of a woman." Another company even claims to help women combat biomechanical issues they face at different times during the menstrual cycle. Thus far, it's been tough or impossible to support their success in independent research studies. There are some studies showing that women's feet are shaped differently than men's, and some studies saying they are the same. Tests we conducted in our lab on running gait when barefoot showed small differences in the location of the center of force in the foot between males and females. But introducing a shoe—not a woman's specific shoe, just *any* shoe, mostly nullified any small differences that we saw.

Almost every other year, some shoe insert company comes out with yet another product that "fixes a women's wider Q-angle." The Q-angle is based on your pelvis, knee, and lower leg alignment. While it's true that women have wider Q-angles, insoles just can't impact this. To "fix" the Q-angle, the insole would have to be strong enought to physically break the leg, completely realign the bones, and then fuse them together again. Is any manufacturer making an insole that does this?

I'm not a woman, but I have a wife and a daughter, and frankly, I've had about all I can take from the folks in advertising. I mean, do any of the differences between men and women *really* make it harder to be a female runner? Lots of individual studies have said lots of different things, but when you compile the data and look at a metanalysis of all the info, only a few things really stand out.

- **Weak glutes**—In general, women tend to have weaker hip stability than men, especially in the frontal plane. This means that the hips are more likely to dive in to the inside in both straight-line running and cutting. Unfortunately, this also predisposes you to various injuries. But don't fret, ladies! The research shows great success with improving your hip strength. You get stronger and have fewer injuries. The majority of women runners should add supplementary hip strength into their training plan, regardless of injury history.
- **Women are more lax**—Women need to deliver a big baby through a very small cavity. This is no small feat! To allow this, women's musculoskeletal structure is more lax. This is a polite way of saying that the joints have more slop or instability. There is absolutely nothing wrong with this at all. Motion is OK as long as you can stabilize it. And that's the problem right there. On the whole, women don't do as good of a job of coordinating their movements as men. This means they are always walking the line between injury and injury-free. If you've learned nothing else in this chapter, remember everyone can make huge improvements in control. Do a better job of controlling the range you have and you'll be fine. Or maybe just go buy another pair of pink running shoes. I mean those advertising folks have to feed their kids, too, you know.

Closing the biomechanical sex gap only takes a few minutes a week. Work on your stability and your "problem" is solved. Problem solved. If only fixing the glass ceiling were this easy, huh?

Summary

There is a method to the madness. Dynamic strength comes in three steps:

1. **Make the muscles smarter**—train the stabilizing muscles to improve coordination and skill during running. Again, high forces through unstable levers lead to disaster. This is the most common problem with respect to running injuries. Get control first.
2. **Make the muscles stronger**—improve the force you generate. Want to run faster? You need to generate more force. When you have control, it's go time.
3. **Spring**—optimize the speed of energy transfer with high speed Olympic lifts and plyometrics.

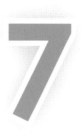

The Footwear Wrecking Ball is Swinging Back Hard, Folks—Don't Let It Smack You in the Head!

A long time ago, man roamed the earth. And then man realized that covering his foot was a good thing. And some other man named Bowerman made the first competition running shoe. And somewhere down the line we wound up with big heavy shoes that are filled with new technology each year. It seems each yearly revision is *more stable* with *more support* than the last year's version to *fix* and *stop* foot motion. Oh, and it also has more "cushioning" than last year's, too. More of everything! The "wrecking ball" of shoe design swung powerfully to the right.

But now, for the first time, runners are firing questions back at the industry. Unless you are a hermit running solo in the wilderness, you've heard the barefoot movement coming into full swing. Several studies comparing barefoot to traditional shoes reveal that shoes significantly alter gait styles and result in tangible differences in gross forces on the body and individual forces at the joints. Chris McDougal's best-selling book *Born to Run* has raised awareness in both runners and nonrunners. The barefooters (most of whom are *not* clinicians) are screaming loudly: "Shoes are evil! Ditch your shoes! Go barefoot 100 percent of the time always for everyone! Barefoot running will save the world!" This type of ranting is just as useless and unfounded as the state of modern day shoe construction.

So let's put the truth out there in the open for both sides to see. Despite many opinions to the contrary, research has shown that today's typical cushioned motion stabilizing shoes are *not* effective in decreasing injury or improving performance. They have not lowered the 82 percent injury rate among runners. Barefoot "tribes" are gobbling up this research and spreading it like gospel through the books, the Internet, and even tattoos. They are grabbing hold of the imaginary wrecking ball of shoe design and fiercely swinging it back to the left. Watch out! Hopefully this ball won't make it too far. Why? There is also *no* research to show that barefoot running decreases injury or improves performance either.

Instead of getting wacked in the head, let's stand back and give it some room to settle. Let's talk about finding a safe spot where we escape the hype and discuss what we know and don't know about shoe design. Unless you are the type of person to kick your friend in the shins, we are all in this together folks. One hundred percent all the time for everyone doesn't always work out.

The Foot: A Self-Identity Crisis

One thing we can all use is some self-confidence. It's hard to have self-confidence if you feel like you've been labeled. Most runners carry around their label like a scarlet letter. They've been told they are a "supinator" or "pronator" and cringe when they expose this mark to their friends. However, you really shouldn't be ashamed. After all, the person you are talking to likely has no clue what you are talking about anyway (and you likely don't either). This situation is ridiculous. Are you scared of the dark? Let's turn the lights on and talk about what all this mysterious foot language means.

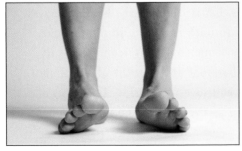

Supinated feet

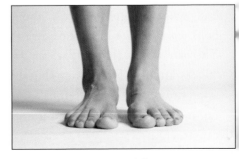

Pronated feet

The foot is a marvelous structure of twenty-eight bones. Some of those bones are weight bearing, and some of those bones are suspended through the four different arches that make up your foot. One of those arches, the *medial longitudinal arch*, is the most prominent one that we see on the inside of your foot. Just like the arch in St. Louis, it has points of contact at the base and something suspended in between. But while the arch in St. Louis was designed to be rigid, the arch in your foot is different.

Arches in the foot are designed to move. Key structures inside the foot passively and actively guide this motion as you stand, walk, run, and jump. This constant state of transition occurs not in one specific joint, but throughout the foot. To keep things simple for point of discussion, we'll focus mostly on the points of contact: the forefoot and rearfoot.

At contact, the forefoot and rearfoot are more or less locked out and aligned in a supinated position. As the foot is loaded, the rearfoot twists on the forefoot. This twisting motion unlocks the foot and allows the arch height to drop. Pronation is actually a very *good* thing. It serves two functions:

1. **Natural shock absorption mechanism**—Think of your arch as a leaf spring in a car. As it "flexes," it spreads out the force. What would happen if you stopped the leaf spring from moving? You'd get a very rough ride! Trying to passively "stop" the foot from moving is not a good idea. All the increased stress from lack of motion will be passed up the body. Runners who supinate stay on the outside of the foot. This keeps the arch overly stiff which passes increased stress up to the shin where we see higher incidence of tibial stress fractures.

2. **Get the big toe down to the ground**—While you have lots of muscles in the foot, the big toe provides about 80–85 percent of the primary support. To provide this support, it obviously has to be on the ground. Once on the ground, the muscles that keep it stable must do their job. More on this in a second.

Active Arch Support

The arch doesn't plummet to the floor and bounce up on its own. While the joint surfaces and plantar fascia provide passive guidance for this motion to occur, the foot is under active control. Specific muscles inside the foot,

Controlled Movement of the Arch

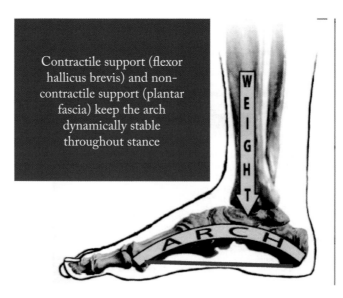

Contractile support (flexor hallicus brevis) and non-contractile support (plantar fascia) keep the arch dynamically stable throughout stance

While forces from above are trying to collapse the arch, you have structures in your body designed to keep the foot under control. If a deficient flexor hallicus brevis (FHB) does not produce tension to stabilize the arch, increased strain is transmitted across the plantar fascia. This is the typical mechanism for plantar fasciitis, as well as a host of other lower leg injuries.

especially the big toe, are at work to keep things in check throughout the twisting and untwisting.

Try this: Grab a hammer and try to drive a nail through a piece of wood. Tap, tap, tap away. Not too hard, right? Now, hold the hammer with your four fingers wrapped around the handle as usual, but with your thumb off the handle and out to the side. You'll notice that you can barely control it. If you strengthened your four fingers, it wouldn't matter much. You need the thumb to come across and stabilize the hammer. What does this have to do with your foot? During pronation, support from the big toe actively stabilizes the twisting of the rearfoot on forefoot. During supination, the toe locks the foot out to create a rigid lever for push-off.

Traditional exercises given to strengthen the muscles in our feet are marble pickups and towel curls. There is a fundamental problem with this approach. The muscles that "curl" the toes originate up in the shin and don't improve your ability to drive the big toe "down" for stability. Doing exercises that provide no specific benefit is useless. If you want to improve the stability of

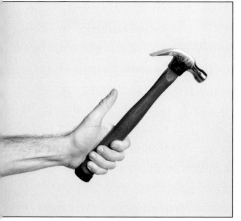

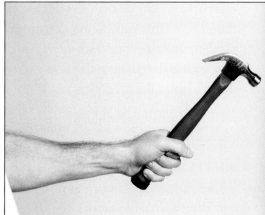

Both the thumb and the big toe dramatically improve your stability.

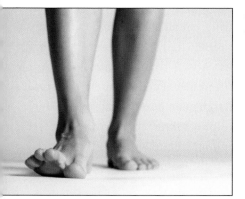

the forefoot, you need to be able to "wrap your thumb around the hammer," or isolate the muscle that controls your big toe. This muscle answers to the name flexor hallucis brevis (FHB). In Chapter 9, we'll evaluate the coordination and specific muscle memory in your foot.

Foot Types

Eyes are different. Hair color is different. Feet are different. Variability is normal. But what really is a *normal arch?* Thirty years ago, if you reported to the Army with "flat feet," you'd be sent home. The misconception is that flat feet can't tolerate the stresses of running. We need to ask a simple question: Do feet that *look* different, *run* differently?

It's always nice when the industry tries to simplify things. Putting everything into separate boxes makes everything nice and tidy. Our long-standing beliefs have told us that very high arches move very little during gait, while flatter feet with collapsed arches move more. You've been "assigned" to a foot type (or cult) and feel safe among your peers. Well, it's time to get out of your box. Research has shown that the trying to "classify" a runner's arch height doesn't really describe what is happening when you run. Differences between structural arch heights are muted when running. Our research has shown the biggest difference in arch movement from stiff feet to very mobile feet is within 1.9 millimeters. There just isn't that much difference between the movement in different foot types. The whole paradigm of *overpronation*, or *moving too much*, just got blown out of the water.

Why isn't there more of a difference? Active control means parts don't just crumple to the ground when loaded. A healthy foot, even a more mobile one, has muscles working both prior to and during contact. Prior to contact, muscles adjust the position between the forefoot and rearfoot to prepare for loading. During contact, muscles keep motion within a very tightly controlled window. "Different feet" *run* more similarly than differently. Further, numerous studies have shown that assigning shoes based on arch type doesn't improve performance or decrease injury. So grab the hand of a runner with a different arch type than you. Sing "Kumbaya." No matter your alignment, we all need to dissipate shock during pronation and actively stabilize during push-off. This job belongs to your foot, not the shoe.

What Happens When Things Go Wrong

Although different foot types move more similarly than they move differently, there is more to it than the amount of motion. Different foot types have different injury patterns.

If you have been called a *supinator*, you stay more towards the outside of the foot and have trouble getting your foot down to the ground. Stiff feet aren't the best shock absorbers and stay more rigid throughout stance. In fact, we see higher rates of stress fractures in the shins of these runners since they can't take advantage of the leaf spring that is built into their mobile arch. They can benefit from self-mobilizing their foot. Grab a LAX ball and roll away on the underside of your foot under full body weight. You aren't doing this for a massage, but to create some movement for shock dissipation within the foot. Another tip that helps these folks is to focus on landing softer. Check out Chapter 8 for more on adjusting running form.

At the other end of the spectrum, we have feet that have been labeled *overpronators*. These people literally think they are doomed, but there is nothing to be scared of folks! Sure, runners with increased mobility have been shown to have more incidence of shin splints, Achilles tendinopathy, and stress fractures in the tibia and metatarsals. But it's *not* because they move too *much*. This is why the term *overpronation* is just not accurate. Mobile feet have problems because the muscles controlling the twisting of the rearfoot on the forefoot are behind the ball. They do activate, but too late to control the twisting of the rearfoot on the forefoot. Muscles inside the foot have to activate and establish a foundation before the bigger muscles can fire. Déjà vu? Does this sound like the core example mentioned in the last chapter? Yes. High forces through unstable levers lead to breakdown.

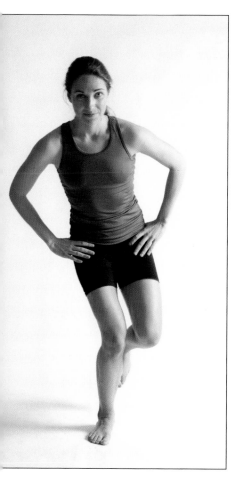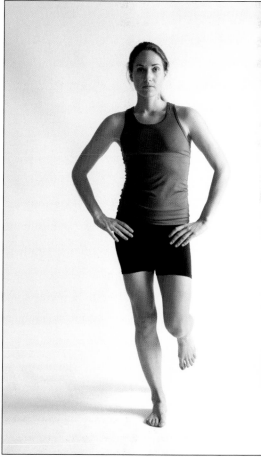

The entire leg rotates in and out with the foot during pronation and supination.

And it's not just about the foot. Ever hear the song "The Hip-Bone-Connected-to-the-Leg-Bone"? The body functions as an interconnected kinematic chain—all the parts influence motion at other parts. The entire lower body moves inward and outward as the foot pronates and supinates. The take-home part here is that things like weak hip stabilizers can actually create excessive motion at the foot. And poor foot control can likewise provide an unstable platform for muscles above them.

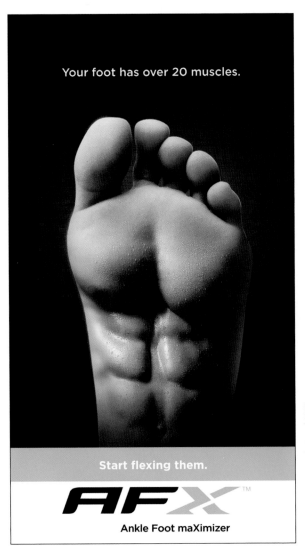

We keep coming back to the idea that the body needs to be controlled as it moves. The concept of "core" stability isn't just for the spine. Improving stabilization of the muscular structures that support and stabilize the foot is important as well. AFX makes an innovative foot-strengthening device to do just that, and their marketing folks developed a picture so powerful it needs no further explanation.

Shoes don't stop the arch from moving and they don't improve the tim-
ng of your muscle control. *This is your job.* The good news is that this is easy
o identify and correct. Check out the "toe yoga" and single-leg squat tests to
letermine where your weak links are.

- Pronation is a natural shock absorption mechanism and increases contact of the forefoot to achieve stability in stance.
- Specific muscles resupinate the foot into a rigid lever for push-off.
- The movement of the foot between these stages is guided and stabi-
  lized by muscles inside the foot, specifically those that drive the big toe
  down for stability and support in stance.
- Any limitations in the foot muscles doing their job can be identified
  and corrected. Do not expect the shoe to improve the activation of
  muscles inside the foot or control the position of the foot.
- Staying excessively lateral on the foot can create shock absorption issues. These runners need to ensure they have enough motion to move
  correctly and can benefit from gait cues to minimize the rate of loading
  (see Chapter 8).
- Excessive twisting of rearfoot on forefoot is the driving mechanism
  behind most foot and lower leg and injuries. The focus for these foot
  types is active stability training.

Surface Variability and Movement Variability

If you train "X" miles a week, why do you have problems in your running
skill? The running pattern is very repetitive and constrained. The literature shows
that some variability in running mechanics is actually pretty good. You have more
than one exact way to put your foot down each and every time. Your nervous system is refined enough to make microcorrections if you land wrong in the steeple
or just running down your driveway. Too little variability means you have no "plan
B." We see this a lot in newer runners. Maybe you felt fatigued during a race, had
to resort to drastic compensations in your form to finish, and were left with an
injury. Too much variability is another common problem, often seen in runners
with back pain and ankle instability. This person can run a lot and may even be
doing lots of core and weight work; however, the way they move is just all over

the place. They don't have consistent strategy to control their movements. Imagine a kindergarten class with zero rules in place; about the only thing you can expect is chaos. It just doesn't work.

It's widely reported that running on trails is softer for the foot and can help reduce injuries. Well, there is actually zero evidence to show that softer surfaces decrease injury. However, there is a significant amount of clinical evidence that shows runners who spend time on trails have fewer injuries than runners who stick to roads. So what's going on? By nature of the rocks, roots, and drops on the trail, running on unpredictable surfaces is more variable than the road. Even though you are just out for a romp in the woods, your body is subconsciously practicing different strategies for foot and ankle stabilization and contact patterns. Mix up your surfaces and you'll refine your skills.

Insights on Traditional Running Footwear . . . Is This the Right Direction?

Your friend wants to hook you up with his roommate. What's the first thing in your mind? What do they look like? Well, research tells us that our obsession with looks carries over to our shoe preferences as well. Consumers overwhelmingly purchase shoes based on looks. Looks are important, but hopefully, you get to know this person before you throw a wedding. How does shoe treat you? What's their personality like? Just like long-term romance, with shoes, "It's what's on the inside that counts."

Traditional construction is fairly standard among brands. While looks are the number one reason you buy your shoes, the second most important reason is "first feel." A great first impression as you slip it on usually means you'll walk out of the store with it. If the shoe feels overly "different" at first step, you'll likely be less inclined to buy it. This makes shoe manufacturers pretty reluctant to make major changes in their footwear design. They want their shoes to feel *better* than others, but not too *different*. Over time, traditional running shoes evolved to share four basic key features:

1. **Postings**—dual-density material that tries to stop motion
2. **High heels**—heel is about two times as high as the forefoot

3. **Cushioned materials**—softer surfaces designed to absorb impacts
4. **Narrow toe box**—narrow toe boxes supposedly improve fit and control

Posting

The shoe industry has adopted the position that its motion control and stability shoes feature *posting*—different density materials on the inside of the shoe—that stops the foot from moving too much. Maximum pronation occurs just after midstance, *after the heel has left the ground*. This means that the posting under the rearfoot that is designed to "stop" the foot from moving isn't even in contact with the ground to do something at the time at which it's theoretically most needed.

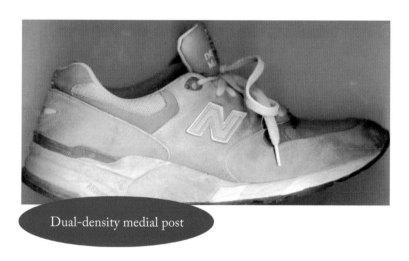

Dual-density medial post

Additionally, these postings create some significant issues at midstance. Even though the foot doesn't stop moving in the face of the medial post, the firmer material means that most runners allow the contact point to drift far to the inside. As the point of contact shifts over the firmer density material, the forces traveling up from the foot also shift. This lever arm now increases stress on the inside of the knee by a significant amount, in some cases as much as 38 percent. Unfortunately, this is one of the main mechanisms for the development of osteoarthritis of the knees. Posting doesn't help and may in fact be causing problems.

Footwear's Effect on the Knee

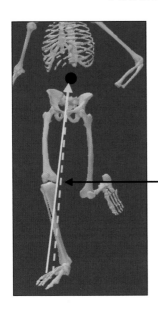

Medial posting increases the lever arm (dashed line) compared to where it normally is (solid line). The increased distance between the knee joint center and the ground reaction force increases the shear force across the knee.

High Heels

Shoes have gotten to a place where everyone—yes, even you, manly men— running in high-heeled shoes. How did we get here? The best explanation I've ever gotten on this goes something like this. Thousands of years ago, shoes were made of very supple materials and were basically like sandals. As tooling evolved over several centuries, people began want- ing more "sturdy" shoes. Wood and crepe were used a lot, but these materials didn't flex much. The shoe was like walking around with a two-by-four strapped to your foot. So cobblers began elevating the heel and rounding the forefoot to make a *rocker*. The shoe could roll off a bit easier and felt more natural to walk around in. Well, that cobbler had a son, and

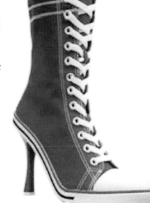

High heels in running: Looks ridiculous, right? So does conventional shoe construction's design with the rearfoot height twice as high as the forefoot.

a grandson, and a great-great-great-great-great grandson who now works at _____(insert name of some major running shoe company here). This way of creating shoes just became the norm.

Now it's well known that the first pairs of Bill Bowerman customs and Asics Tigers were flat. But over time, heel heights moved back up. Why? While this is just me speculating, it's probably a combination of two things. First, most folks walked around all day in shoes that had high heels, so most people were more used to the Achilles and calf working in a shortened position. Second, raising the heel allowed running shoe companies to fill this area with more technological "stuff" to cushion the foot. Was this really necessary? Or just the way things were? Who knows? But it's where most of us have wound up.

Is an elevated heel a good idea? Well, let's look at this from a human, not a shoe, standpoint. No matter if you believe that man evolved from caveman, was divinely created from Adam and Eve, or blew up from a dust particle (The Big Bang, anyone?), there is no record of caveman, man, or dust running around in a pair of stilettos. How's that for being politically correct? The foot should be flat. My friend and colleague Dr. Mark Cucuzzella has a good view on this. He says: "The null hypothesis is that the foot works best when flat." In science, the null hypothesis is the accepted thing that you try to disprove, and until it's disproven, it continues to be the thing we assume correct. Studies have shown that elevated heels compromise foot proprioception and throw off normal muscle firing patterns in runners. And yet, no one has shown that a flat foot position is a *bad* position to be in.

So should we all be 100 percent flat, 100 percent of the time? The proprioceptive responses of the foot works best when flat. If your feet were flat most of the day, it would be like secret training. Think about how much of your day you *aren't* running. If you put your foot in a better position all day long, you'd be able to maximize your foot function. Remember—multiple skills carry over in multiple activities. Even if you aren't running in flat shoes, it's a good idea to try and get in them during work or school. There are several dress shoes out on the market that are flat yet look good enough for the office.

Cushioned Materials

Modern running shoe construction is filled with revolutionary materials reported to cushion and stabilize the foot. These shoes absorb mechanical loads and offset work that the foot must do on its own. While this sounds great in theory, there is a point of diminishing returns. If your friend holds you up as you run each and every mile, eventually the muscles in your body will weaken since you've become dependent on that friend for support. Cushioning has changed how our foot responds to the running surface.

The foot is the direct contact point between the ground and the body. Just like all the other parts in the body, it works best when it receives good sensory information on where it is and what position it is in. Nerves that conduct proprioceptive information are large and well insulated, making them the *fastest* relay system in the body. Firm surfaces provide good feedback to determine the position of the foot. If there is a delay in getting sensory information to our brain, there is a delay in stabilization from the big toe. With stance periods as short as 0.07–0.25 seconds, this muscle response must be strong and quick. Anything that delays this signal is fighting you.

Overly cushioned materials between the foot and the ground "filter" this sense of feedback. Don't get it? Try this. Tie your shoes. Not that big of a deal right? Now, tape about 50 marshmallows on your fingers and palm, and then tie your shoes again. Which is harder? All those marshmallows prevent you from feeling the laces and make it really hard to use your fingers. You feel clumsy and uncoordinated. Sticking the foot inside a marshmallow (an overly cushioned shoe that is ramped up at a 2:1 ratio above the ground) impairs muscles from rapidly correcting foot position throughout stance. If a foot gets vague

Marshmallow Midsoles Impair Feedback

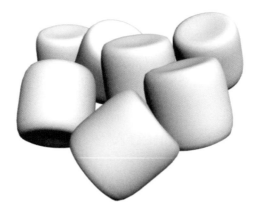

information, it produces a vague response. Less filter means more feedback, more muscle activity, and more control.

○————————————○

Narrow Toe Box

Your foot is basically a lever, and compared to our height, it's a very short lever. A wider foot has more leverage and therefore more stability. Take a look at a newborn's foot. You'll notice that the widest part of their foot is not the ball of the foot, but the toes. Since about 80–85 percent of foot support should come from the big toe, a slightly wider big toe dramatically improves leverage. Your body was born with good alignment.

Unfortunately, almost everyone reading this book has been practicing the ancient art of Chinese foot binding. Fashion has dictated that we have shoes that taper in the front. This has caused our big toes to move inward, dramatically decreasing leverage from the big toe. Compare the foot X-rays in typical running shoes and in a pair of wide toe box minimal shoes. You'll see that the toes are squeezed.

What effect does a narrow toe box have? Poor position equals poor function. It's really hard to activate muscles if a joint is pushed in one direction over the years. While the *flexor hallicus brevis* drives the big toe *down*, the *abductor hallicus* widens it to improve leverage. If you can improve control to drive the big toe down and actively spread it, you'll experience true Zen in foot control. But it's tough to learn this with a foot that's had a vice grip on the toes since you put on your first pair of shoes. So the first thing we need to do is get into shoes with a nice wide toe box so the foot can splay.

Dr. Ray McClanahan is a podiatrist in Portland, OR, who is big on prevention. Instead of trying to "fix" the foot with surgery and orthotics, he first tries to get the foot to work better on its own. He shared his simple shoe fit test with me, and I'll share it with you. When you are shopping for shoes, take out the insole, put it on the floor, and stand on it. Since standing on your foot widens it, the shoe should not constrict this natural mechanism stability. More foot splay = more leverage = more control. If you look down and see your foot hanging off all sides or the top of the insole, it's not the right size. You want your foot weight-bearing on a consistent surface. Shoes that taper aggressively through the arch (like most running shoes) constrict the foot and compromise

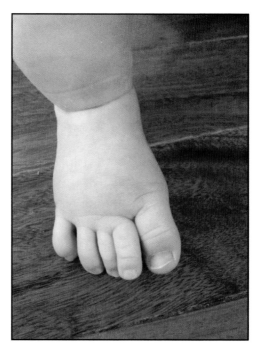

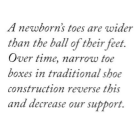

A newborn's toes are wider than the ball of their feet. Over time, narrow toe boxes in traditional shoe construction reverse this and decrease our support.

position sense since some of the foot is weight-bearing on marshmallows and some of it is on the upper mesh. A wider shoe allows your foot to work the way it was designed to.

A lot of barefoot and minimal runners say that their foot is getting bigger. There is nothing to be concerned about, and this may even be a good thing since a bigger base is more stable. Running shoes should be about function, not fashion. Adjust your size if your foot grows.

The take-home: Traditional running shoes have changed the position and behavior of our feet. While people can bicker back and forth about technicalities of footwear research, there is an underlying and somewhat disturbing message: Despite all the technological advances over the years, traditional shoe construction (featuring heels twice as high as the forefoot, with cushioning and pronation control devices) has not resulted in decreased injury rates or improved performance in runners. Codependency really isn't a good thing.

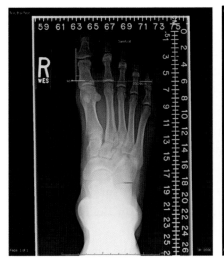
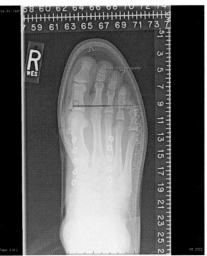

Chinese foot binding? I'll let these X-rays speak for themselves. Take a look at the natural splay of the foot when barefoot. Now take a look at what traditional toe boxes do to our foot. Not a pretty picture, is it? Squeezing your foot puts the squeeze on your foot control.

The phone rings. It's you asking me to design your T-shirt for the next 10K race your club is hosting. So I start the design for the T-shirt on my laptop. Later you drop by and we move the file to your superfancy laptop. Your computer is nicer than mine, but the quality of the design is still relatively the same no matter what computer it's on. You aren't happy with my layout (hey—I'm no designer!) and decide to call a professional graphic designer. She shows up with her five-year-old laptop and presents an incredible design that you love. You could care less what kind of computer it was produced on, right? You didn't hire a computer, you hired a designer. What in the world does this have to do with shoes?

We have this idea that we are dependent on shoes. We go shopping hoping to fit into a shoe. Umm . . . excuse me. The shoe works for you, not the other way around. Sure, shoes do make a difference, but a pair of shoes has yet to win Boston unmanned. You are the skilled professional operating the shoe. Take charge of your foot and the shoe will follow.

Do I Need Orthotics?

Individualized custom orthotics are commonly used as part of a comprehensive treatment plan. Numerous studies show success after using them, with "success" defined as symptom reduction. Orthotics are used to help align the joint around which we pronate and supinate. They claim to "control movement," improve the stimulation and proprioceptive response, and improve biomechanical efficiency. Sounds just like some of the shoe research, right?

Let's cut through a lot of the research and deal with what orthotics really do. Orthotics are a very powerful tool to tailor a contact surface to a runner's individual alignment needs. A clinical assessment of the foot (outside the scope of a book like this) is needed to determine if there is a structural alignment problem. One of the goals of pronation is to get the big toe down to the ground. If the runner has a structural alignment issue where they cannot get the big toe down or cannot get it down without significant compensation elsewhere in the foot, they are likely an excellent candidate for orthotics.

However, orthotics are overprescribed. If the runner has good structural alignment, I'd rather them use the $300 for a weekend getaway with their wife or maybe textbooks. Instead of spending money on the magic pill, spend time to stabilize the foot for a long-term fix. Simply sticking something in the shoe makes the foot dependent on the orthotics and actually makes the foot weaker and more dependent on the orthotic. If you've made it this far without them, there's a good chance you don't need them. If you have them and want freedom, there is likely a chance if you can get your foot working up to par. Talk to your local clinician and see what best matches your individual needs.

Is there anything that can actually help my foot work better?

Want to look hot for your date? It's time for a "mani and pedi," guys and gals. That's right. We are going to spread those toes out just like they do when you hit the spa for your pedicure. Above we mentioned some muscles that are critical for stabilizing the big toe (we'll assess these muscles in Chapter 9). Physically spreading the toes makes it much easier to "find" these muscles. Dr. McClanahan has created an innovative product called "Correct Toes" to do just that. The difference between Correct Toes and the foam toe spreaders from the spa is that Correct Toes are flat on the top and bottom. You can sleep in them, wear them at work all day, and you can run in them as well. (Again, make sure your toe box is nice and wide to allow your forefoot to splay.)

What will these do? Spreading the toes does three things. It improves the leverage of the forefoot, optimizes position of the big toe to improve muscle activation, and also keeps tissues in the plantar fascia mobile. These attributes are beneficial no matter what kind of foot you have.

Who should be a bit careful with these? Runners who have significant bunions (hallux vagus). While you look down at your foot and see that the big toe points inward, that's not really the source of the problem. By definition, hallus valgus occurs when the bone upstream from the big toe (the metatarsal) shifts outward. Correct Toes won't have any effect on the alignment of this bone, and in fact may actually create an issue. How do you know if they are for you? I use this test for people with bunions. Move your big toe out laterally as far as you comfortably can, then extend it up to the ceiling and hold it there for about 20–30 seconds. If this is uncomfortable, it means that you are compressing the joint surfaces. If this is the case, I'd skip them. If it feels OK, fashion your own toe spacer out of duct tape and wear it between your first and second toes for a few days. If all goes well, order up a pair.

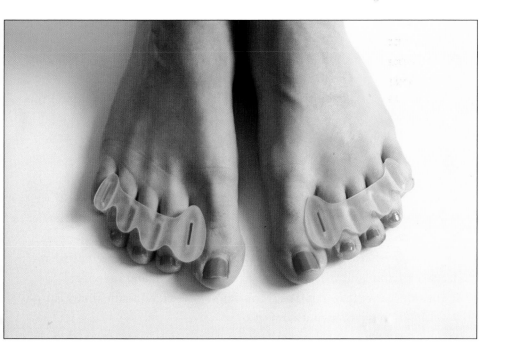

While there are no long-term independent tests on this product, I wouldn't let that scare you too much since the long-term tests on shoes don't really help us out much either. (An unorthodox approach? Yes.) Most footwear products are marketed to stop or support the foot when wearing them. Correct Toes are one of the few products designed to improve the foot when wearing them, as well as improving coordination even when you are not. If you are someone who has trouble with the toe yoga, balance, and stability tests, they can make the difference between "I have no idea how to control my foot" and "My foot is so stable it feels like a steel I beam." Both personally and professionally, I'm a big fan. Check them out at *www.nwfootankle.com*.

Do You Know What You Don't Know?

Sometimes things sound really nice. Things that sound nice make us feel warm and cozy. Traditional lore passed down from coaches, retailers, the shoe industry, and even clinicians is based on the idea that we should "stop" and "stabilize" the foot and that feet need cushioning to protect our bodies. In fact, five to ten years ago I was teaching and publishing based on these same traditions that had been passed down to me. I helped clinicians match foot type to shoe type to help each foot get its specific blend of motion control, stability, and cushioning. Didn't we all but dispute this already?

Guess what. If you think you are done learning when you get your degree, you are sorely mistaken. Research in the past few years has shown that our previous understanding of footwear prescription is based on well . . . traditions as valid as smashing freshmen on the head with a ring (common practice at my high school; all it does is get you in trouble).

Shoe research is a big buzz topic right now. There is a lot we know and a lot we don't know. The shoe community is just figuring out what it doesn't know, and it is targeting research, clinical, and individual case studies to see what works for certain runners in certain situations. For now, the investigation continues . . .

Going Nude: What Happens When You Take Your Shoes Off

The barefoot buzz is big and oftentimes very obnoxious. But to ignore some very interesting work coming out would be just as narrow-minded as saying that conventional shoes are best for all runners. You'll never pin me down to say that barefoot running is "better" than traditional shoes. True barefoot running is different. And when I discuss barefoot, I mean 100 percent barefoot. No minimal and no five-finger shoes allowed. However, there are some very important lessons to be taken from barefoot gait that apply to everyone's gait.

Barefoot runners don't just run with their shoes off, they run *differently* with their shoes off. Several studies comparing barefoot to traditional shoes reveal that that shoes significantly alter gait styles. Traditional shoes with a squishy high heel mask our foot's sensation and allow us to land hard on the heel well in front of our center of mass. This overstriding can let you become "sloppy." This sloppy form does a number of things that increase the mechanical stress of running and compromise efficiency. No matter what you have on your foot, overstriding is not a good thing. And then you practice this sloppy form for 10–120 miles a week. Ouch.

Running barefoot eliminates the "filter" between your foot and the ground. All this extra *feel* helps you bias your gait style into a better form. For a detailed look at what barefoot running does to your running form, check out Chapter 8. For now, I'll spill the beans: the changes in form you experience while running barefoot are much more powerful than anything you do or don't strap to your feet.

Is Barefoot More of a Drill or For Real?

I can't tell you exactly what to do here. At the least, running barefoot is a very functional drill. The foot is a sensory organ—give it some sensation that it doesn't get while wrapped up in a smooth sock inside your smooth cushioned shoe. Getting out of your shoes and doing some barefoot drills is a really great way to practice feel and position sense. This whole book is about mastering athletic skills to improve you as a runner, and this is just one more way to improve your skill set. If you love it and want to up your volume, go ahead. The whole reason you are doing this stuff is because you like it, right?

Foot Strength—I Noticed You Didn't Say Much About That—Doesn't Barefoot Help This?

Remember the strength chapter (Chapter 6)? We outlined the paradigm of *stable* leads to *stronger* leads to *quicker*. Sans midsole, there is considerably greater demand on the muscles in your foot. Over time, you can gradually improve your foot strength. However, I'd think about this more practically. If you want rapid improvement in the muscles that help you run, you need to do more than just run. The strength chapter should have instilled in you the idea that you need to specifically target your deficiencies. The best way to strengthen your foot is to strengthen your foot. Do lots of single-leg balancing and get out that medicine ball and rocker board to boost the challenge.

I Want to Try Barefoot Running. Will It Hurt Me?

When barefoot running hit the big boom, some "experts" warned we should brace for a windfall of new injuries. They claimed that barefoot runners would have fewer instances of certain injuries while increasing other running injuries. While there are reports of case studies here and there of barefoot runners getting hurt, there are also case studies of runners getting hurt in shoes. One survey from our lab asked 518 barefoot runners if they got a "new injury since they began barefoot running that resulted in them needing to seek clinical care." Only 6.7 percent of respondents said yes. No, I'm not thrilled that 6.7 percent of these folks got hurt. But since 82 percent of runners get hurt anyway, such a small number of runners getting hurt is kind of like doing another study asking how many folks got hurt running in a red T-shirt. Historically, runners get injured. As long as you use your brain and progressively increase your volume, barefoot running doesn't seem to be causing the widespread rash of new injuries that many feared, and it may have some benefits.

Are There Any Other Drawbacks to Barefoot Running?

I'd say there are two issues here. First, running over rocks on the trail and drug needles in the city is no fun. My coworker, Corey Rynders, joked one day that he could stop the entire barefoot movement in one fell swoop. He wanted to collect bacterial and fungal cultures from the foot of a barefoot runner following a tromp through the city. Once people saw all the the dirt on their feet and likeliness for open cuts and scrapes, barefoot running would quickly die out. This is obviously a far reach, but the point is simple. If your local running grounds aren't conducive to tossing the shoes, don't feel like you are failing; protection is always good.

The second drawback is where things get interesting. The barefooters have been claiming that because they don't have to haul the weight of a shoe around, they are more efficient. Well, this is actually false. The foot works *more* when running barefoot. While the increased proprioception and foot muscle activation is great for injury prevention and running form, there appears to be somewhat of a metabolic cost to running barefoot. Compared to running in shoes, you'll expend 3–4.5 percent *more* energy to run barefoot at the same pace.

Times They Are a-Changin'

You aren't alone in trying to find better shoes. The shoe industry is scrambling to keep up with the fastest growing market segment. Almost two years ago I gave a talk at a medical conference on new (at the time) research on barefoot running. At that time, there were only six "minimal" shoes on the market. One year later, there were sixty-four. Numbers like this don't signal a passing fad.

And much more has been going on as of late. The industry is realizing that motion control shoes are not really controlling motion and have been scaling back their volume in this segment. They are being forced to ask a simple question: Did we evolve the shoe for a specific reason, or did we evolve it because the tech department gave us some cool materials to play with and we had to have a new three-letter acronym to sell at next year's shoe review? Good things are coming out of this. One of the major companies has even gone so far as to drop the heel heights on almost its entire line. The word is spreading. The focus is moving away from *stabilize and cushion* and more towards *don't screw up natural foot function*. While the shoe construction pendulum is stabilizing, it's tough to say exactly where it will settle.

The industry has embraced this new thinking as *minimal* footwear. However, the current definition of minimal footwear is certainly grey. The combination of the slope of the footbed and its height off the ground leads to a number of combinations. You may find a shoe that is 100 percent flat but higher off of the ground. Another minimal shoe might have a ramp from forefoot to rearfoot, yet be closer to the ground. And still another might be completely flat (called zero-drop) and only a few millimeters off of the ground.

Decision Time: What's Best for Your Foot

As an athlete, you are focused on improving your engine, and now (!) your chassis. For starters, the best shoe for you may be the one that you are already in. Despite everything we've said above, there really is no mind-bending evidence for me to say that you have to ditch your current shoes if they are working for you without any problems. That's not to say that changing couldn't make things better (or worse!).

However, if you are looking at something to help you improve as a running athlete, there is mounting evidence to shift our previous tendencies in shoe design. Traditional shoes aren't decreasing injuries or improving performance. Running barefoot has many advantages for the body but is not practical for most and it will impair your performance economy. Some recent studies have shown that lightweight shoes are actually more economical than going barefoot. Yes, *any* shoe is heavier than barefoot, but having a lightweight, minimal amount of shoe between you and the ground decreases metabolic work in the foot while providing less interference with normal foot function for injury protection.

So what does this leave us looking for? An ideal shoe looks much like some of the first running shoes ever created. They should be:

1. **Thin** – A little protection goes a long way.
2. **Firm** – Just enough midsole to optimize proprioception in the foot, minimize work of the foot, but not so much to allow hard landings in front of the body.
3. **Light** – Weight matters for efficiency.

Shoes don't set PRs. Shoes that result in *positive responses in the body* are beneficial. You want enough to protect the foot and let it work. Anything else is a waste of your hard-earned dollars.

Where should you begin?

Currently, your foot is adapted to high-heeled, cushioned shoes with a pronounced rocker from the heel to the forefoot. Making small changes in the shoe geometry and construction can be made easily with little impact to your training plan. Making a large jump to a zero-drop shoe or barefoot will take additional time and adaptation. So how minimal should you aim for?

How far to drop depends on your individual needs. If adjusting the training volume and intensity is not an option based on your current training plan, the move can be much more gradual. A good rule of thumb is to start with half the distance of your current shoe drop. If your current drop is 12 millimeters, moving to one that is 6–8 millimeters results in considerably less impact to your body and training volume than a more aggressive drop. As your body adapts, the end goal will become clearer for you. Some will find that getting to 100 percent flat is where you are happiest, and some will find that you are happiest at 3 or even 6 millimeters. Failing to get to zero drop does not mean you've failed. You are investing time to improve the function of your foot no matter what is laced on your foot, and you've found an end goal that is working for you.

During daily standing and walking, go with as little shoe as you can get away with (close to or at zero drop) to demand more muscle activity from your foot. You spend significantly more time not running than you do running. Raising the baseline level of foot muscle activation all day adds up over time. Numerous companies now make flat dress shoes that will pass through all but the snottiest law offices. Throughout the day, try to spend as much time as possible on one foot. It's secret *training*.

How about running? You should aim for the lightest shoe you can get away with considering your current training F.I.T. goals, and internal mobility and stability. Going to zero drop is an excellent move to minimize the lever arms acting on the body and is an excellent long-term decision for runners with arthritis, degenerative joint changes, compartment syndrome, and loading rate problems during gait (see Chapter 8 for more on this). A minimally cushioned flat shoe lacks a compressive midsole and can significantly reduce the tendency to overstride.

Comparison of Shoe Styles and Their Effect

Reason to:	Stick with your current shoe	Transition to a more minimal shoe design 3-8mm heel height with a firm, thin, and light design	Transition to a zero-drop shoe (No height differential between rearfoot and forefoot. Usually have a form-fitting anatomic shape that is close to the foot, yet allows forefoot splay.)
Benefits	If it's working and you have no pain, there is no reason to make a change.	Improved intrinsic muscle activity, improved balance, proprioception, and foot strength. Lighter weight to improve economy.	All the benefits in a minimal drop shoe with the addition of minimized lever arm on the joint at all cost. Highly effective in runners with arthritis and joint degeneration, compartment syndrome, runners in need of decreasing their loading rates.
Impact on current F.I.T.	None.	Drop current heel height by ~half (typically 6mm). Begin with half volume in this shoe for 2-4 weeks. Following this period, continue volume as normal.	Very gradual transition: wearing the shoe walking around for 2-4 days. Initial run is a half mile. Increase volume about ¼-½ mile each run thereafter.

Transitioning to Barefoot and Minimal Footwear

Ditching the rockers and squishy stuff in the shoe requires a little bit more from your foot. These tests, all described in detail in Chapter 9, offer a simple way to see if you have what it takes for a safe transition:

1. **Mobility test** –Tests ankle dorsiflexion and big toe dorsiflexion to ensure you have enough motion to roll over the forefoot.
2. **Foot control test** – Through big toe stabilization, it tests isolated control of the big toe.
3. **Stability test** – Through single-leg balance, it tests balance and proprioception of intrinsic foot muscles.

When your foot "works," it moves enough and actively stabilizes the transfer of forces through the foot. If you don't pass these tests, don't worry—get to work on improving your limitations. If you lack mobility, direct your efforts towards improving your soft tissue length and tissue mobility until you pass. Remember, stretching will take ten to twelve weeks to gain significant improvements and soft tissue mobility will take about three weeks. If your limitations are in the balance aspect, you'll be amazed how quickly this improves if you simply practice, practice, practice. Typically, about two weeks yields a significant improvement. Finally, strength gains take about six to eight weeks to achieve.

Passing these three tests doesn't mean that you should go run a marathon in your new minimal shoes on day one, but we've seen that folks who master these have little to no problem making the transition. Please note that these tests are not only for barefoot hopefuls; all runners—even those who run in traditional shoes—should pass these tests. However, with the traditional shoe construction you've been accustomed to out of the picture, your body has to have a bit more going for it to make up the difference.

How Many Shoes Should You Have?

Ladies, this number cannot be infinity! Some runners run in one pair of shoes. Some runners rotate through two to four pairs a week to let the shoe recover from a workout. Gang, shoes don't have feelings. They don't take a day or two to feel better about themselves after you stomp all over them. Running physically breaks down the midsole of the shoe. It doesn't rebound or bounce back. A three-mile run and a four-mile run always adds up to seven total miles on the shoe no matter how many days came between the runs. There's no problem with rotating your shoes, just realize that it's not to extend the lifespan of the shoe.

Is there another reason to have more than one shoe? I'm going to have to say yes. Road and mountain bikes are better at different things; shoes can be good at different things as well. We've harped on the point that soft squishy materials impair foot control. Getting to as minimal a shoe as you can get away with will eek a bit more internal muscle control out of your foot. I spend every day in zero-drop minimally cushioned shoes at work, play, and for most of my easy runs. I am building up my foot control all day, every day. Secret skill practice! But if I'm looking to do a serious workout, the focus is on my engine. Even though I can run fast in my flat shoes, a bit "more" shoe allows me to concentrate on going hard and using less effort to keep my foot in check. I'll grab a pair of shoes that have a 3–5 millimeter heel and weigh about 6-7 ounces.

Some conservative runners may read the above statement and say—*Yes,* that's *exactly* why the typical 2:1 heel height is better—it offsets more work by the body! However, this is untrue, unproven, and allows a runner to adopt a suboptimal contact style. In the future, there may be better or different ways of matching shoes to runners on the grand scale. For now, we can only provide what we know. Due to the controversial nature of shoe prescription, a list of shoe references is available in the appendix. In the future, we may have more concrete information on exactly where the pendulum should stop its swing, but for today, the best we can say is to select the right *thin, flat,* and *light* tool for the job and make sure that your *foot* is in the driver seat.

"But It's For the Kids!"—What Is the Best Footwear for Your Children?

Take a look at the American Podiatric Medical Association guidelines on children's footwear and you'll see something that doesn't make sense. It states: "Select a child's shoe that's rigid in the middle. Does your shoe twist? Your shoe should never twist in the middle." Then written in fine print, there is this statement: "This does not apply to toddlers' shoes. For toddlers, shoes should be as flexible as possible." OK, two-faced Joe, which is it? Stiff or floppy?

I've had the privilege of working with some African runners. These athletes were born without shoes, and ran, played, hunted, and harvested crops without shoes on. Back in the anatomy chapter (Chapter 3), we discussed that soft tissues and bones remodel based on the way they are loaded. Going barefoot throughout their rapid growth periods in the first two decades placed more mechanical load on their foot than the typical American kid wearing blinking light-up marshmallows. What is the result? These folks developed with strong, stiff feet. Shod societies have foot problems that the unshod world does not have. Plus, your infant already has excellent foot alignment. The widest part of their foot is their toes, not the ball of the foot; that's something to consider.

I have a four-year-old and a toddler. I want them to develop strong and stable feet. It's a small choice I've made for them to improve their parts. Do I have stacks of independent peer-reviewed data to back up my claims that unshod societies have better feet than shoed societies? Nope, and I could care less. After being simply blown away by the straight big toe alignment, incredible foot strength, and stability of runners who grew up sans traditional footwear, I'm sold. No foot binding for my kids for as long as I can control things! They will never be in a narrow shoe or one that doesn't pass my flex test. What is the flex test? Hold the shoe between your thumb and forefinger. If I have to "try" to bend the shoe, it's too stiff. Kids are light, and a little bit of stiffness goes a long way. I've been given traditional kid shoes by family and friends, and I politely send them to Goodwill.

I know it's not cool to tell other parents how to raise their kids. I'm only giving you something to think about. Right now there aren't many minimal kids' shoes out there, but hopefully this will change in the very near future. Just as the barefoot studies are raising eyebrows in adults, I'm hoping parents will see that this information isn't exclusive to them. The goal is to develop a strong stable foot for life. I don't want the shoe to get in the way of well-rounded development for my kids: barefoot as much as possible and as floppy of a shoe as I can find for everything else.

Summary

- The traditional paradigm of shoe construction has proved that it does not achieve its goals; it has not decreased injury rates and it has not improved performance. The gait patterns that these shoes allow us to get away with aren't usually the best option.
- Barefoot gait results in beneficial changes in gait to preserve joint health while somewhat negatively impacting economy.
- Shoes don't stabilize the arch. Muscles do—train 'em!
- Good shoes help our foot work better. *Better* would be defined as improving your stability to decrease injury risk, optimize performance, or bias you into a better running form.
- Minimal shoes, with a firm, thin, and light construction and a wide toe box appear to be the optimal criteria to allow maximum foot function and protection.

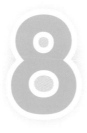

Essentials of Running Gait—The Human Slingshot

When you were a kid, you probably did fun stuff. Some time or another you probably shot a can off a fence with a slingshot. It's simple really. Hold the slingshot, pull back on the elastic band, aim, release and—*whap*! Rock hits the target. You probably didn't give much thought to what was going on in the slingshot; you were more focused on the target. Your brain did a bunch of precise calculations to figure out how much to pull back, where to aim, and how to release to get the best trajectory of the rock as it flies through space.

I'm lucky to work in a gait lab with well over a million dollars of toys. It lets me analyze some very specific and very complex stuff in runners. We stick reflective markers on the runner just like they do when they digitize movies and video games. This lets you see how much someone moves when they run. Most runners freak out and get excited when all the dots move all over the screen. In reality, all it represents is how much they move. Sure this is important, but even more important is "*why*" a runner moves they way they do. We use other special equipment to measure the forces acting on the whole runner and each individual joint. Sounds complicated? Actually, it is.

But let's reverse the norm. Instead of looking at running and making it more complex, let's do the opposite. Let's take all the fancy data we get and make it simpler. And then we'll make it simpler yet. I'm going to propose a model simple enough for Grandma to understand, yet comprehensive enough to help the gurus out there make sense of all the little trees they've heard about. The next time you hear or read a piece of advice, think about how it fits into a paradigm we'll outline here. Your body is a human slingshot, and I'd like to help you hit your target.

To achieve this "Holy Grail" of running form we must admit something; there is a *lot* we know about running form, yet we still have much to learn. To determine exactly how *you* should run after conducting an individual one-on-one assessment is actually quite doable. If you know what you are doing, it's pretty easy to provide specific information to a specific person to optimize their body and running form. However, it's a bit tougher to describe how everyone should run. People aren't rocks shooting out of a slingshot. They are a system of pulleys and levers, muscles and tendons that move those parts, and a brain to process and refine the reflexes and control the limbs. Even with all this variability, good running form should play by a few rules. Optimal *running economy* would emphasize as much speed as possible by using as little energy as possible.

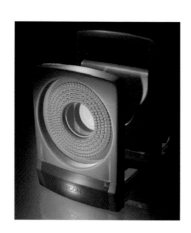
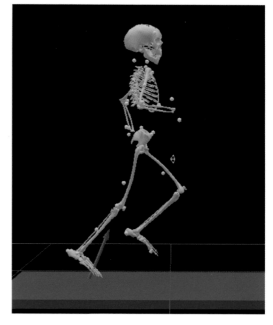

Special cameras let us visualize the dots to determine motion (dots and the corresponding skeleton), while force plates measure the external forces acting on the runner (the red arrow). Understanding what those forces do has the greatest impact on your economy and injury risk.

Your Invisible Friend: Elastic Recoil

It takes a lot of energy to move the body. Even standing requires some amount of energy. Walking requires more energy than standing, and running requires even more. Muscles generate the energy needed to let us stand, walk, and run, but wouldn't it be cool if your muscles didn't have to support all the energy demand? If something else did most of the work, your muscles could reduce their contribution, and your economy would improve. Fortunately there is! In fact it's not just a minor help, it's a pretty big one.

The main energy source we use when running comes from the storing and releasing of elastic energy. If we have good storage and release of elastic energy then our muscles don't have to work as hard. If we store too much or can't release properly (two of the most common problems in runners), our muscles have to do more work to keep you running along.

When running at a steady speed, your foot contacts the ground in front of the body, so from the point of foot contact until the foot is directly under the center of mass, you are in an *energy absorbtion* phase. Most folks call this the *braking phase*. Even though this is totally accurate, we are avoiding this

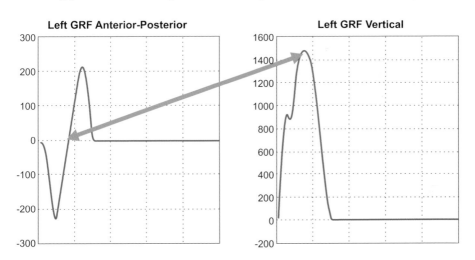

At contact the foot is in in front of the body, and the body stores elastic energy inside the tendon. Note the negative values on the A/P curve on the left. At midstance, the foot is directly under the body mass and counters the high vertical forces. No storage or release of elastic energy is taking place at the exact time of midstance. From midstance through toe-off, the A/P GRF (ground reaction force) curve shows energy is released from the tendons to drive the body up and forwards. Note that every single runner has some type of push-off, irrespective of what gait style they use.

terminology right now because runners get bothered by the idea that they might be braking when they are running. In fact, some of these new proprietary running styles have told runners that they should minimize braking at all costs and land directly "under their body." While minimizing braking forces sounds nice, it's not exactly true. To run faster you actually need to store energy in the loading phase so you can release it later.

Unless you are accelerating, your foot *always* lands in front of your center of mass, and in fact this is a *very good thing*. The whole point of landing in front of your body is to store elastic energy. Some of this "free" energy is stored in the vertical direction, and some of it is stored in the horizontal direction. If you struck directly under your body, your muscles would actually have to work very hard and produce more energy, at a greater energy cost to you. The slingshot can't fire a rock unless you load the band with tension. You'd have to just pick it up and throw it yourself, which requires more of your own energy. But the slingshot makes it easier to launch the rock. *Contacting in front of the body stores energy inside of the tendons, just like pulling back on the rubber band stores energy in the slingshot.*

Once you've reached midstance, the foot is directly under the body and the ground reaction force is at its peak. To counter the force pushing you down, your muscles need to have enough multiplane stability to keep the parts stable.

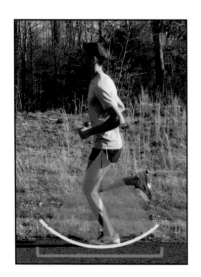
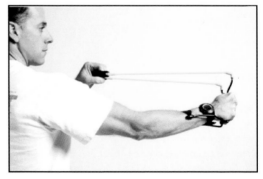

You store energy in the slingshot so that you can release it to fire the rock. This is the same thing we do when running. We store energy from contact to midstance, and then release it from midstance through push-off.

Storage (red) and release (green) of elastic energy

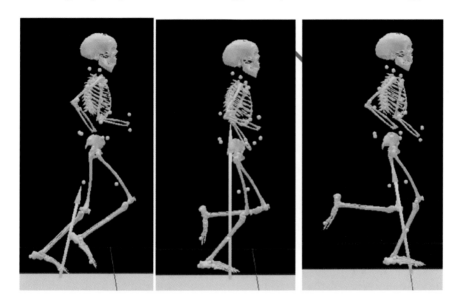

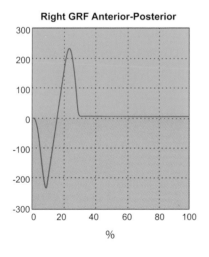

Right GRF Anterior-Posterior

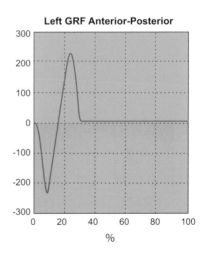

Left GRF Anterior-Posterior

If you didn't have enough dynamic control to keep things stable, you'd lose elastic energy transfer. Let's say that the hip dives to the inside during stance due to weak hip abductors. In an ideal world, muscles don't change length when running. However, the weakness in the lateral hip muscles makes them lengthen. The transfer of energy from the tendon is impaired and requires extra metabolic work to stabilize the hip. If the muscle excessively shortens or lengthens, it costs extra to run the same speed. To repeat what's been said many times throughout this book: High forces applied through unstable levers lead to disaster. Revisit the slingshot. With the band fully loaded, it takes more effort for your lead arm to hold the base of the slingshot stable than it does when unloaded. If you can't keep the slingshot stable, all that wobbling around is going to make it tough to hit your target.

So we've stored energy into the body, are keeping it dynamically stable, and are ready to *release*. From midstance through toe-off, we do just that. Your muscles are working. They are producing just enough force to keep things stable, but the majority of the force lifting the body up and forward comes from the tendon. One note here, some of the trendy running form folks say that you should avoid "pushing off." Let's take a quick second to separate the unicorns from horses. One hundred percent of all runners in any gait lab, using any gait style imaginable, will register a propulsive force 100 percent of the time. Everyone pushes off using recoil. Release the band, and the rock goes flying.

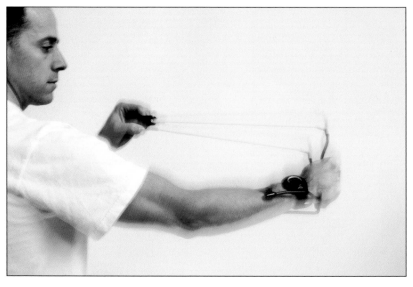

If the slingshot isn't stable, you are in trouble. Refer back to the stability chapter to fix these issues.

So How Much Energy Should You Store and Release in Your Human Slingshot?

This has to do with your speed and your *pendulum*. One more analogy to tie this all together: a grandfather clock. The pendulum on the clock sways back and forth in an arc around a pivot. If you push the pendulum in one direction, you store energy in the pendulum. When you release it, this energy causes the pendulum to swing to a given point on the other side of the clock. If you want to increase the arc of the pendulum, you have to use more force to push the pendulum. So a small push produces a small arc of the pendulum, while a large push produces a larger arc. Similarly in running, it all comes down to the pendulum.

The arc that the foot scribes beneath your body is similar to a pendulum. It contacts a certain distance in front of the body and should toe off roughly that same distance in back of the body. How big should the swing be? *For a given speed, the runner who has a "tighter" arc in relation to the body is more efficient than the runner who has a larger arc.* Why? Doing is always better than reading. Try this little experiment:

- **Exercise 1**—Stand right in front of a set of stairs with your toes touching the bottom of the first step. With one foot on the ground, place the other foot up on the step in front of you. Without leaning forward from your trunk, step up on the stair in front of you.

  Lever arm – The farther away the force is applied from joint center, the more muscles have to work. For a given velocity, contact closer to the body with a tighter pendulum. As the swing of the pendulum (your leg) increases, the lever arm increases and the body has to travel up and down more, which cost lots more energy.

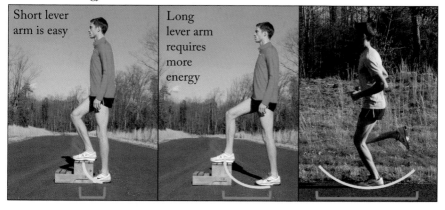

Short lever arm is easy

Long lever arm requires more energy

- **Exercise 2**—Repeat this same step-up, except this time, you are going to stand about one foot away from the first step, and without leaning forward from the waist, step up.

Which is tougher? For those of you too cool for school, I'll tell you the answer, but you really should try this to help make it stick. Exercise 2 is harder. When you put the foot further in front of the body, you increase the distance of the contact point (foot) from the pivot point (effectively the center of the pelvis). This results in a larger *lever arm*. The greater lever arm, the more muscle force you need to raise the body.

When running, a foot that contacts farther from the body also means there will be more up and down motion of the body and more slowing down and speeding up during the stance phase. All this extra change in momentum is not necessary and is less economical for a runner. Your limbs should be kept straighter and closer to the body to minimize energy expenditure. Obviously, the arc scribed by the foot will need to increase as speed goes up, but the rules still hold true. Overstriding is not economical.

Flying Through the Air

How much of this energy release shoots the body up and how much shoots it forward? Ideally this depends on speed. Go grab a slingshot and a rock. Your mission is to shoot the rock as far as possible. Do a little experimenting. Pull back as far as you can and aim high in the sky. The rock will launch superhigh in the air, but when it returns to earth, you'll see that it didn't really cover much distance. Most of the elastic energy was spent on fighting gravity. Remember that gravity is pushing down on you with about two and a half times your body weight when running. It costs much more energy to raise the body up and down than it does to cover horizontal distance. As of right now, there are no style points given at running races. Excessive up and down motion of the body actually wastes a lot of energy that you could be using to run faster.

Which requires more energy: running 5 percent faster or running up a 5 percent grade? Think about it. It's harder to lift up a piano than it is to slide it across the floor. Raising the body up and down against that crushing 2.5 times body weight challenge is the most taxing aspect of running. In fact, holding the body up against gravity accounts for almost 80 percent of the energy you expend while running. This is why running up hills is much harder than just running faster.

So does this mean you should minimize your up and down motion? Let's shoot another rock. This time we are going to aim very level. While the rock doesn't go very high, it likely goes a little further. It didn't have much time to travel forward. Go for a short run and keep your head as still as humanly possible—it takes a lot of effort! Steps that are too short waste energy.

Grab another rock. Let's really try to maximize distance on this last attempt. Aim higher than level, but not too high—aim somewhere in the middle. Release! The same amount of elastic energy was transferred to the rock in each situation, but this time the more optimal angle allows you to cover much more ground with the same effort.

How much up and down motion should you have when running? If the body was a simple rock, a high school physics class could answer this question easily. The general answer is that your body should move up and down about 1.5–2.3 inches (4–6 centimeters), and this depends on speed. But it also depends on a lot of other things as well. Runners aren't just rocks; they are complex creatures that do things during their time in the air and time on the ground. Everyone has different structural and neuromuscular restraints that limit us from making blanket statements about all runners. Small changes here make a big difference. The person who nails this is on their way to a Nobel Peace Prize. Get on it.

Timing

What the body does when running and *where* it contacts are both related to how *quickly* the whole cycle takes place. The research on the speed of our contact cycles is based on the time of contact with the ground, and while cadence and stance time aren't exactly identical (you can run with a long hangtime and a short contact time and vice versa), it's a bit easier for runners to understand since cadence is easily measured.

Then what is an optimal cadence for runners? Is it this magical 180 that everyone talks about? Anything that causes muscles to change in length compromises transfer of our "free" elastic energy and increases metabolic cost. Hanging out on the ground for too long moves the body up and down a lot, which changes muscle length and wastes energy. This is frequently seen in recreational runners with a cadence of less than 160 steps per minute.

Should stance times be short? You'd think so. Common sense dictates the longer you spend on the ground the slower you are traveling. Coaches have overwhelmingly jumped on this bandwagon as they seek to reduce stance time as much as possible. Counter to this predominant thought, this is *not always optimal* either. There are no studies to show shorter ground contact times are better, and there are studies that show shorter ground contact times are worse. When ground contact times decrease, internal force to lift the body upwards and forwards must be generated even quicker. If contact time is too short to achieve "rebound" of the stored elastic energy, additional fast twitch muscles step in to close the gap.

Sprinting is taxing because the ultrafast contact times required mean you can't "wait" for the elastic rebound to be released. Muscles must supply incredibly high forces, producing rapid fatigue. But a sprint race is over very quickly. Who cares if they are fatigued after? The emphasis is on power, and economy is rarely a limiting factor. However, for distance runners, this increased fatigue can be the difference between standing on the podium or falling to the back of the pack.

So where did 180 steps per minute come from, and is it an old wives' tale?

Coach Jack Daniel's observational research claimed that 180 steps per minute was an optimal running cadence. This was based on watching runners and not really testing any characteristics of the body that would affect this number. However, a recent experiment did look at the optimal *recoil time* for shortening and lengthening of tendon. Jumping with a frequency of 3 Hertz (three times per second) produced the least metabolic energy expenditure and the best exchange of elastic energy. Jumping with a frequency less than or more than 3 Hertz, utilized more energy cost. Interestingly, three contacts per second multiplied by 60 seconds yields 180 contacts per minute. This is not to say that everyone should adopt 180, but it does give us a physiologic rationale why this may be a good starting point and provides our "U-shaped" economy curve.

Efficiency versus Speed

Real world performance data has seen races won in virtually every distance with a range from 178–235 steps/min. Truth be told, there isn't a lot of good data examining the effect of cadence on metabolic economy. A look at a older cycling study poses an interesting paradox. Cyclists were tested to find the most efficient cadence. Any guesses what it was? Very low—it was in the low 40s! Remember, economy is maximizing power output with as little energy

nvested as possible. This is likely why most folks spin easily around town on
. beach cruiser with low cadence. However, no one has ever won the Tour de
France with cadence this low. Professional cyclists develop massive amounts
)f power. They need to average between 300–450 watts with spikes over 1,100
watts. The priority is *not the most economical zone*, but the generation of more
)ower for more speed. Enter the *pain cave*. Sure, efficiency matters, but the
vhole game shifts in light of the demands of the peleton.

The gravity-dependent nature of running obviously introduces different
factors than cycling, but this trend is still likely in effect. The only way to
un faster is to increase stride length (distance per stride) or stride frequency.
Although increasing cadence above the "U-shaped" *economy curve* may not be
he most efficient strategy, it may be a necessary one to run the times that
vin races and break records. Is there anything you can do to minimize the lost
·conomy at higher cadences? *Yes*—elasticity can be improved through train-
ng. Doing high intensity lifting and Olympic lifts can help stiffen the neu-
·omuscular system so that you can decrease stance times with less of a ding in
·our economy. If you are a competitive runner and still lifting high reps of low
veight, it's time for a shake up in your weight room training. Check back to
Chapter 6 for more.

So where does this leave us with respect to cadence? There is no *single*
ffective cadence for everyone. Differences in genetics and training impact
ndividual elasticity and likely account for a lot of the variability seen on the
ace course. This being said, *stance time should be as long as possible without
·inimizing the effects of elastic recoil.* Research shows that both too long and too
·hort of a stance time increases muscle work. Be realistic. If you are a highly

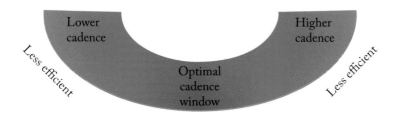

*In individual's true optimal cadence is likely at the bottom of their "U." Increasing or decreasing
·he cadence from this point typically negatively affects economy. This needs to be examined as part
·f the equation since running faster may require going past the point of economy. Likewise, cadence
·odification can result in significantly less mechanical stress to the runner with only a slight ding to
·fficiency. Intense strengthening and time spent training these other cadence rates can minimize the
·ing on economy.*

competitive runner at the national and international level, it makes sense to utilize higher cadence as a tool to improve performance. Cadence is a variable that can and should change somewhat with speed. However, I'd be hard pressed to say that a midpack age grouper should run around 220 rpm. Likewise, runners who are significantly lower than 90 rpm at comfortable and tempo paces would likely be well-served to increase cadence by 5–10 percent to experiment and observe changes in economy over the long term. We at least need to help get most folks on the radar—towards the bottom of the "U-shaped" efficiency curve. Appropriate rise and fall of the center of mass is important to maximize recoil and likely occurs around 90 rpm, and can be modified by differences in a runner's unique elasticity. Metronomes are excellent training tools to cue this skill while running.

Check out recoil yourself.

Try to do ten fast, light jumps in succession like you would if jumping rope. Feels rather "springy" doesn't it? Now jump a few times in a row again, but do it very slowly. Squat down pretty far, jump up to max, and then squat down again. Takes a lot longer to do the jump and feels quite a bit harder, right? Slower movements limit our ability to use this "free" elastic force to move our body. If you want to be your own lab rat, try the following experiment. Download a free metronome program on your Smartphone, and set it to 180 to start. Jump up and down on each beat for about 10 seconds. Then adjust the tempo of the metronome up and down slightly and see if you find a zone where it feels easier to jump at the rate of the metronome. Do you feel the "U-shaped" curve at work? Likely you'll find some rate between 170-190 that feels easiest for you.

- Our human slingshot helps us run efficiently.
- We run by storing and releasing elastic energy.
- Good dynamic stability improves the exchange of this "free energy."
- Failing the stability tests in the assessment section likely means you are expending more energy than you need to at a given speed.
- The foot should scribe an arc that is tight to the body for a given speed.

- Enough rise and fall of the body in both the stance and flight phases is optimal; too much or too little compromises efficiency.
- Optimal stance time should be as long as possible without minimizing the effect of elastic recoil. For most runners this is around 180 rpm.
- Efficient cadence for most is likely self-selected. For most runners, this is around 180 rpm.
- Sometimes efficient does not equal the fastest (in the quest for speed) or best (when musculoskeletal issues are a concern).
- Changing cadence can have large biomechanical effects on decreasing energy absorption on joints, particularly at the knee.
- Runners near the high end of the performance window should train to improve their muscle stiffness to minimize losses in economy with the high cadences they require.

How Do You Screw Up a Good Thing?

Elastic recoil is yours for the taking; use it. But what if your chassis has some issues? Specific limitations in your body compromise your ability to run efficiently. If you happen to be taking notes in this book, I'd circle this, then star it, and then write it on your fridge so you can see it every day, and focus on each limiter until you pass the test. Specifically you need:

1. Enough motion to get the leg behind your body (the backside of the pendulum)
2. Postural stability
3. Strength and power of the gluteus to drive the body upwards and forwards

Mobility and Its Effect on Your Pendulum

As mentioned previously, speed is dependent on stride length and cadence. Your stride length should be symmetric with equal swing in front and in back of the body. Again, imagine the pendulum of the grandfather clock swinging back and forth equally. Every runner I've ever seen can get their leg in front of their body just fine. They don't have problems on the "front side" of their pendulum. But a lot of runners have mobility restrictions that prevent their pendulum from swinging through on the backside of the body. Thus to achieve the required stride length for a given speed, *the oscillatory path (or swing) of the pendulum is shifted forward in space.* This completely alters the storage and release of elastic recoil mentioned above. Vertical rise and fall of the center of mass (COM) is increased, approach and departure angles are increased, energy absorption at the knee occurs, and elastic recoil is compromised.

What Structures Are Typically at Fault Here?

Deficient motions to get the leg behind the body:

1. **Tight hip flexors**—Due to the predominance of sitting in Western cul-tures, the majority of the population has tight hip flexors. These tight hip flexors limit your ability to extend the hip while keeping the back in neutral. To an untrained eye these runners do get the leg behind them, but they do so by arching the back, not extending the hip.

Running in the Backseat— trouble getting your leg behind your body

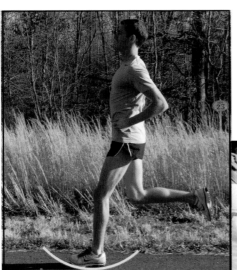

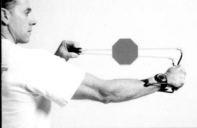

Store energy OK, but can't get release
Arc of leg shifts in front of COM

- Typically from tight hip flexors
- Also from restricted talocrural and 1st MTP (metatarsophalangeal) mobility
- Core deficits and postural weakness are common in this running form

2. **Limited mobility of the ankle and big toe**—Normal ankle dorsiflexion is between 35–40 degrees, and normal dorsiflexion of the big toe is 80 degrees. You don't need this much to run. You need a little less at the ankle and a lot less at the big toe. However, most people measure the motion at the big toe when the foot is nice and relaxed on the exam table. This doesn't show what happens when running. During running, the lower leg rolls over the ankle and all the slack is taken up in the muscles in the calf and Achilles tendon. The only structure left to elongate is the plantar fascia. If it's tight, you won't be able to get the essential 30 degrees of dorsiflexion when the toe is loaded. Just like the hip flexor limitations, your push-off is cut short requiring your pendulum to shift forward in space.

Shifting the path of the pendulum limits the release of elastic energy. Let's look back at the slingshot again. Imagine pulling back and then letting go. But instead of transferring all that stored energy to the rock, your mobility restrictions are like a wall that stops the release of energy halfway. You stored all this energy but can't take advantage of it; it's like putting on the brakes.

Since the pendulum can't swing behind you, stride length reaches a limit. To increase speed, cadence must increase beyond optimal, and as mentioned prior, these shorter stance times lead to decreased efficiency.

This shifted pendulum doesn't make any friends with those of you with chronic knee pain. Since the pendulum must swing farther out in front of the body, there is a larger lever arm and thus more load on the knee. Normalize symmetry of the pendulum and you'll get an instant decrease in load on the knee and typically knee pain as well. Want to know if you are in the clear? See the mobility assessments. Roughly 80 percent of you have limited hip extension. Ouch. And although less of you will have limits in big toe motion, you still need to check. Just because you don't have a history of plantar fasciitis, it doesn't mean that you have enough motion in the plantar fascia.

Postural Stability

Poor core control *shifts the pivot point* of the pendulum. When the lumbar curve increases, the center of mass moves back with respect to the foot placement. Thus foot contact occurs further forward of the COM and energy absorption increases. This increased energy absorption doesn't pay off, though. Instead of getting released, it gets dissipated through the body. Go check it out in real life. Watch the 1,500 meters or the mile. Picking out which runners have good or deficient control is easier than deciding what to watch on your satellite TV. For the first three laps, you'll typically notice excellent postural position for the entire pack. Then watch what happens to the field over the last 300–400 meters of the race. In virtually everyone, the lumbar curve increases and the pelvis tilts forward in space. This change in postural alignment is associated with an increase in metabolic effort to maintain speed. Thus when trying to put forth your best effort over the final lap, the efficiency of the runner is actually decreased. Not a good race plan! For more of this, check out the core section in Chapter 10.

Let's put it in even simpler terms. Running fatigues the body. Running faster during interval workouts or during races fatigues the body even more quickly, and requires good core muscle control to counter this. Actually, you need excellent core muscle control. Knowing all this, you'd think that developing *excellent* core stability would be something all competitive runners work on daily. Not just planks. Or crunches. Or some type of med ball partner twisty thing.

It comes down to awareness and *feel*. If your perception of good posture is really posture stuck in the backseat, it doesn't matter how much core strengthening you do; you failed. It's OK for gymnasts to finish a vault with a ton of arch in the low back after they complete the exercise. It's not OK for you to increase you arch when running. Know what correct postural alignment feels like. Know what F.A.T.S. has done to our perception of core position (yes—you too guys, and especially you swimmers who live in a pool doing tons of lumbar extension for hours a day). The more time you spend in excessive lumbar curve, the more normal it feels. Instead, you need to feel that you are in fact in correct position at any pace. Uphill. Downhill. Fast. Slow. Practicing correct alignment when not running makes sure you can find it when you are. The more you practice good posture, the easier it will be to maintain it when running. I'd say we've beat this dead horse enough, but because so many of you have trouble with core control and hip extension, we'll keep harping on it until I start seeing people (you!) maintain core position over that last lap. Want to improve elastic energy usage? Work on core control. OK, rant over.

Strength and Power From Hip Extension

As speed increases, more and more power needs to come from the hip extensors: your glute max. That's right. It's all about the booty. A weak glute max sends you down the *toilet bowl of doom*. Why so grim? Well, you know all that posture stuff you just read above? These folks with a weak glute max get a big "F" on all of that plus more.

You have two main muscle groups that extend your hips: your hamstrings and your glute max. However, there is a major difference between what these muscles were designed to do. The hamstrings were designed to move the hip; they are more fast twitch in nature and are not designed to hold any type of postural stability of your pelvis on your femur. The glute is different. It's often said that the glute is the strongest muscle in the body, but is it true? Look how big your quad is compared to your glute. Strength doesn't always revolve around size; it has to do with leverage. The glute max has one of the most direct lines of pull of any muscle in the body. It can generate a *lot* of force to extend your hip. However, the trump card here is that your glute has a higher percentage of slow twitch fibers. What does this mean? It means that your glute max is not only the most important muscle extending your hip, it's also the most important muscle keeping your pelvis stable on your hip.

If you have to move a mound of dirt, do you want to do it yourself, or do you want help from some friends? The way to make *any* sport more efficient is to spread the work around. More muscles under less load is always better than less muscles under more load. Distance runners are not only deficient in using muscles on the back side of the body, they actually train to overwork muscles on the front of the body. Take a look at a sprinter. Sure, they are more muscular than distance runners, and yes, they spend a good portion of their race accelerating. Good sprinters will be able to reach peak acceleration, but the person who wins the race is the one who decelerates the least. Sprinters know they must maintain excellent postural control, and they must capitalize on the incredible leverage of the glute and extend their hips to maintain speed. Isn't maintaining speed a primary goal of distance runners?

What are the most commonly preached drills for distance runners? A-skips and B-skips. Ugh! Why! A-skips and B-skips are both reported to increase elastic recoil. OK, I'll buy this somewhat. A-skips emphasize activating the hip flexors. B-skips are reported to help get the foot moving at the time of contact. Some people call this *pawback*. Let's quickly clear this up. At steady speed, the foot contacts ahead of the center of mass; it doesn't matter if it's *pawing back* or not. The point of contact is ahead of the center of mass and that's that. If you've never heard this term, don't worry about it; it's about as real as a unicorn. Any force graph in the world will show you that from contact to midstance, the foot is in front of the body and the goal is energy storage. Am I saying that I want runners to push back into the ground far in front of them? Of course not! The point is that these drills that emphasize hip flexion aren't really that effective for distance runners.

What kind of runners benefit from hip flexion help? Sprinters, 800-meter runners, and milers under 4:40–4:20, depending on their individual form. Why? These folks are moving pretty fast! You need to be able to get that leg out in front of you and ready for contact. What about the rest of you? In all my years of collecting objective data on runners of all disciplines and abilities, I've never seen a runner who actually had deficient hip flexion strength or recruitment. If anything, I've seen way too many runners who dominate with these muscles. Thus when the runner gets tired, they go back to what they *know*. They try to increase their stride by reaching out in *front* of the body. This shift actually increases energy storage and doesn't help energy release. The runner is less efficient. What's a better decision? Instead of reaching out in front, push off better with muscles on the backside—the glute max. Your body needs balance. Backwards running and heel lift drills should be mandatory each and every run. Regular skipping is a great way to emphasize lift without contacting too far in front of the body's center of mass. Run from the butt, not the quads.

So let's describe the *toilet bowl of doom*. It really is a beautifully engineered screwup of epic proportions. These runners start out with a poor posture. Their hip flexors are typically very tight. Tight enough that their pelvis is cranked forward in an anterior tilt (imagine spilling your cereal bowl forward). On top of this, their glutes are too weak to maintain position of the pelvis above the femur. At some point (it might be right away or might be at mile or ten), they'll fatigue the pelvic position and their arched back and tilted pelvis will roll forward on their hips. As their entire body rotates forward in space on their legs, the center of mass comes forward with it . . . a lot. So far that they'd normally fall on their face.

So what happened to the slingshot in this case? Instead of just pulling back on the end with the rock, let's reach forward with the hand holding the sling base. Go ahead—reach really far out with your lead hand. The first thing you'll notice that you are off balance and unstable. Second you'll notice that it's hard to do this! You are now storing way more elastic energy than you should be, and you still get blocked similar to what happened above. This is about the most inefficient form possible.

Runners with poor posture are forced to overstride way in front of their body to widen their base of support and to avoid falling on their face in front of their friends. This produces a number of compensations in the spine, hips, knees, and ankles. Someone with this gait pattern could tell me any number of their parts hurt at some point in time, and I wouldn't be surprised in the least. Sooner or later with enough F.I.T., the pipe bomb in your toilet is going to blow. What is the efficiency level with this gait pattern? Try dragging an

Toilet Bowl of Doom

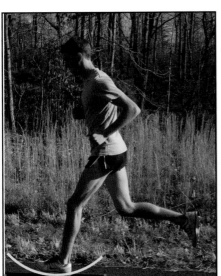

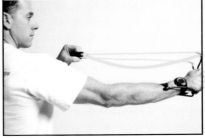

Weak glutes allow the torso to pitch forward. This postural change requires you to step much farther in front than normal.

The runner lands on an overly straight leg with a high loading rate. To combat this, the runner sinks down and flexes the knee more than typical. A lot of energy is stored as the center of mass is lowered more than we'd like. And it takes even more energy to raise the body back up.

anchor alongside you. This form overloads the muscles in front of the body and is exhausting.

Is there a fix? Sure there is! But these folks don't respond to cues like *run tall* and *keep your spine in neutral*. They pretty much have no idea they have a spine, or a hip, or any muscles that control them at all. Their specific muscle control is really inhibited. So where to begin? Begin simple. Start with simple exercises to get the muscles *smarter* and do lots and lots of reps. Every single day. Do it until you know without question that you are doing them just as you should. Build muscle memory first, and then add another and another. And one day a little lightbulb lights up for the first time and you get it. Then you can work on cueing posture when you walk, stand, and even run. Just start simple.

Other Glutes

While we are on the topic of glutes, let's also mention two other muscles that factor into hip control: the gluteus medius and minimus. Their job is to keep the pelvis laterally stable on the femur. While the glute max is a postural stabilizer and a hip extensor, it is also your most powerful external rotator. So all three of these muscles work in concert to keep the hip steady during gait, but there is a simple little visual that can identify which one is most limited.

The force to run comes from the legs. The arms' job is to counterbalance the upper body on the lower body. When you see someone run with a wide arm swing, it's basically a red flag that they have deficient lateral hip stability. It may be on one side or both, but it's a pretty telling clue that there is a major imbalance in lateral control. Other runners may have an arm swing that crosses midline. This is more indicative of a rotational imbalance somewhere in the lower body. Lateral stability problems are improved when you work the glute medius, and rotational control problems are improved when you work the glute max. If you see this dominant arm swing pattern in your gait, fix the limitation in lower body control, and the arms will naturally adjust and counterbalance.

A Big Problem Leads to Bigger Problems

The following points highlight some very common and major weaknesses we see in runners, but it's important to know that each one can cause more than one weakness. Because these key compensations result in dramatic shifts in where forces are in relation to the body, they affect other locations in the body as well.

- Limitations in your body shift the storage and release of elastic energy and increase the cost of running.
- Limits in hip extension and big toe dorsiflexion prevent the foot from getting behind the body as it should and block the release of elastic recoil.
- Postural weakness and increased lordosis also block the release of elastic energy.
- A forward trunk shift combined with increased lordosis dramatically increases energy storage and requires significantly more metabolic work, as well as negatively affecting loading rate (see Chapter 7 for more on this).

The above patterns are not due to a failures in training, but rather due to failure to address comprehensive mobility, strength, and skill development . . . *and are correctable!*

Let's think about a runner with inhibited glute max strength. To run a certain speed requires a given amount of force. Now the glute is a major player in delivering force to the extending hip, but if you can't activate it, force has to come from somewhere. One of those places is the calf. I've seen a lot of runners who have chronic Achilles issues but don't really have major stability problems at the foot and ankle. The problem is actually up the chain. Because they can't get the hips to store and release this elastic energy, their calf is forced to do way more work than it was designed for and breaks down. No amount of stretching, mobilizing, and ankle strengthening will fix this scenario.

In a previous chapter, we said that the best way to make a good casserole is to start with good ingredients. Which kind of athlete will give you the best form? Take a look back to the end of Chapter 6. Hopefully you'll pick the stable athlete with the big spring. Knowing what to do and being strong enough to counter the forces of gait keeps all the forces where they should be. If you aren't this runner yet, don't spend time stressing. Spend time fixing. You don't like it when a co-worker asks you to do things outside of your job description do you? Neither does your body.

Target your issues. Carving out time to fix them is your job. The most targeted way to attack your limits is head on. *Great athletes* aren't scared—they embrace and attack their weaknesses head on. Earn yourself a spot as a great athlete.

Why Are the Elite Runners So Fast?

Elite runners have great parents. I'm not saying that they were loved more than you, but their inherited genetic potential for high levels of physiologic performance is incredible. Yes, they work *very* hard, but so do you. Do you have a medal around your neck from the Olympics? If so— please give a nod to your ancestors. Elite runners have the ability to generate massive amounts of aerobic power, which tends to trump many other factors. Their muscle fiber types are optimal for the events they compete in, their ability to extract oxygen from circulating blood is through the roof, their balanced nutrition provides essential building blocks, they sleep a lot to promote adequate recovery, and they typically have a coach that knows how their body responds and adapts to their training. All of the stars have to align so that an elite runner can make it to the big show.

Gait Form and Injury

Just as we outlined factors that effect economy, we need to outline constraints that affect injury. As we've learned in this chapter, limitations in the body affect running form, but this equation also works in reverse; your form can also affect your body. Changing the way you run either increases or decreases the stress on the body.

It's really, really easy to run with a form that minimizes your chance of getting hurt. In fact, that's the key word: minimize. If all the forces, lever arms, and demand on the body are minimized, there is significantly less breakdown on the runner. Less mechanical wear and tear equals less chance of injury. Less internal muscular strength is needed to stabilize the body. Everything just got easy! All you have to do is run slow with very short strides and a foot landing very close to your body. There is really only one downside. Less stored elastic energy with this gait pattern means less "free" energy. So if you want to run fast with short strides, you'll be taking strides both as short and as fast as a hamster. It's just not very efficient.

This doesn't mean that this is a "bad" way to run; it depends on your goals. Maybe your goal is to run several days a week for long-term fitness or weight loss or maybe just for social reasons with your friends. Minimizing wear and tear is OK even if you sacrifice some efficiency. Your biggest concern is ensuring you can run another day to clear your mind and erase your stress. Or perhaps you are trying to resume running following time off from an injury. You can tell that your strength is lower than it should be and you keep the stress low temporarily until you get stronger. Or maybe you have mild arthritis or a meniscal tear and want to keep running with minimal breakdown of your compromised parts. Running like this sounds like a smart plan actually.

How about those of you on the flip side? You want the PR. You are goal-oriented and set on winning your age group at the local 5K, qualifying for Boston, or landing on the podium at the NCAAs. Speed is critical, but so is staying healthy for consistent training.

While it's very easy for folks to minimize stress on the body when running slowly, it takes *more* from you to run fast. In short, you have to earn the right to run fast. Peak forces in running are a product of body mass and running speed. So the faster you go, the more strength you need to counter these high forces, produce a longer stride length, and increase your turnover. What happens if you can't produce these higher forces but continue to run fast? At this point you are a betting man.

There is nothing inherently wrong with running faster if your body is up to the task, but when fatigue sets in during the race or workout and your form shifts, you start loading the body in ways it was not designed. Maybe some little aches and pains show up. Maybe some minor things become chronic. Maybe something goes past its threshold and results in an injury.

Why throw all your poker chips on red? You know that higher intensity training is more stressful. Plan for it. If you get a plan down, you can have your choice of cake and eat it, too. Yes, there is a way to minimize the training stress on the body even while running fast. It's the Holy Grail of running form. To help explain this, we are going to add in the ever-hot topic of barefoot running.

As speed increases . . .

Forces increase	Higher forces acting on you require increased strength to maintain form and minimize the effects of fatigue.
Stride length increases	Longer stride means that the pendulum of the leg swing must increase. A larger swing of the leg away from center of the body increases the lever arm acting on the joints. Thus, the need for specific muscular stability, especially in the lateral and rotational planes, increases.
Cadence adjusts	Although not as much as stride length, cadence increases slightly to maintain a certain amount of stiffness in the legs to maintain energy transfer.

Case Study

I've been working with a runner who fits a classic pattern I've seen time after time: he instantly biases his posture into lumbar extension the second he gets tired. He says that he does about forty-five minutes of core work every day, and I believed him, so I asked him to show me exactly what he does. Watching him perform all of his exercises, I noticed a common trend. The first thing he does is increase the curve in his low back, overtightens his lumbar extensors, and then does the respective movement for the exercise. This is the exact position he practices every day for forty-five minutes. No wonder he continually faults into increased extension.

So how did we fix this? This runner was doing college-level exercises, but he never mastered basic components of core control he should have learned in kindergarten. I told him to stop his previous core routine and prescribed a series of very basic exercises that he could do 100 percent correctly. He did thousands of reps over the next few weeks trying to re-program his perception of correct movement. As his specific core control improved, we progressed in the complexity of the exercises. Exercises are great, but to really fix this issue, we needed to implement this new muscular control into his running form through drills and cues.

Things were gong very well. His injuries cleared up and his form with base and tempo training was flawless. Then he jumped into some faster level speed sessions at race pace. It was like going back in time. All the compensated postural issues we'd worked so hard to eliminate came back immediately. His core control had improved tremendously over initial levels, but it wasn't good enough to hold him in proper alignment at race intensity. So we adjusted his intensity according to his weakest link. He was allowed to run as fast as he wanted to until his form broke down. We continued to do exercises to trigger the correct neuromuscular patterns, but running with a strict emphasis on maintaining core neutral at high speeds helped narrow his focus. After a few intervals, we would chat and discuss exactly how his muscles and positions were feeling so he could learn how to identify his boundaries.

Fixing postural problems in running starts with making muscles smarter, making them stronger, and most importantly, transitioning this new muscle memory into running form. Close the gap. Fix the form. Run your best.

Loading Rate

Loading rate is the speed at which you apply forces to the body. While running, you aren't going to change your body mass (OK—I know you can slightly due to hydration issues, but let's ignore this for a moment). Your total mass stays *relatively* the same and thus peak forces remain relatively the same. However, *how* you move your body's mass forward when running determines the way your body is affected by the forces we see in running. Loading rate is something we measure in the gait lab. Quite simply, it's the slope of the ground reaction force (GRF). If you look at the graphs on page 169, you'll see that one graph has a steeper slope to it than the other. The steeper slope (top graph) means that the forces applied to the runner occur more quickly than that of the forces applied to the less steep slope (bottom). Why does this matter?

Imagine running fifty miles a week. Think of the amount of wear and tear that occurs on the body. Now imagine running fifty miles a week with a gait pattern that causes the mechanical loading of the body to occur less quickly. Decreasing the loading rate applied to tissues will minimize tissue stress to the runner, minimizing the effects of the microtrauma of endurance training. The rate at which structures are loaded has been implicated in both stress fractures, plantar fasciatis, patellofemoral pain syndrome, and low back pain.

So should everyone lower their loading rate? Just because you have a high loading rate, that doesn't mean you are guaranteed to get one of these injuries. However, anytime you can change a variable of your gait to reduce the causative biomechanics of more than one injury, it's something to consider. But it's also important what you do to decrease your loading rate. Some methods produce a lower loading rate with no detriment to economy. Other styles can lower loading rate while increasing metabolic cost. The goal is to get the loading rate as low as you can without compromising economy.

Then what causes a higher loading rate? Well, let's stare at the proverbial tree of rearfoot versus forefoot just like everyone else in the country. Yes, contact style makes a difference here. In general, runners who land on the forefoot have a nice gentle slope, while runners who land on the rearfoot have a steeper slope. No argument there. This has been published extensively and something that I can validate in my lab in less than a minute. This is like adding extra shock absorbers to your car; it helps spread out the load between two joints instead of one. However, trying to minimize the loading rate with only a forefoot contact won't lead you to the Holy Grail. Why not? While landing softly on your forefoot typically results in a decrease of your loading rate, it actually increases energy cost. The few studies that have compared the metabolic cost of barefoot running to lightweight shoes all find that the lightweight shoes are more efficient. This means that something beyond shoe mass is at play here (since there is no shoe mass at all in barefoot running). There is likely a "cost" associated with stabilizing the forefoot. On some occasions, a strict focus on forefoot contact produces very large shifts in economy. In our lab, we call these large shifts the "the prancy fairy." (It's not a put-down—this is literally what these folks look like—almost like they are running on hot coals.) They do successfully lower their loading rates, but they are very inefficient. To be fair, these runners most typically also have hip extension limitations that force compensations in lumbar posture. The take-home message is that the tree representing forefoot contact doesn't hold all the answers.

So what is up with that other 10 percent of barefoot runners who land on their heel? While this may sound odd, they've learned to land *softly* on the heel and closer to their center of mass when running barefoot. This brings up an interesting point: There is *zero* evidence that a heel strike is bad for you or anyone else. Yes, I've heard all the folks running around saying that everyone should land on the midfoot, but it's a little inaccurate as well. And even more odd, we occasionally see runners who contact on the forefoot but have high loading rates. Hmm, landing on the forefoot explains much of the truth but not all of it

Loading Rate and Contact Styles

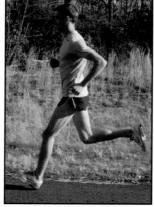

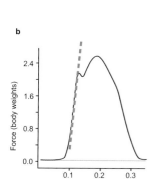

Typically, contact styles that feature a heavy heel strike far in front of the body produce a steep loading rate, while contact styles that occur on the forefoot and midfoot closer to the body result in a less steep loading rate.

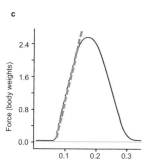

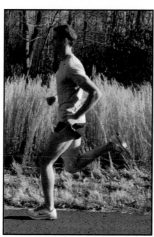

Barefoot running results in more than just a change in forefoot contact. It also changes stride rate, stride time, and where the foot contacts in relation to the center of mass. Ninety percent of barefooters contact on the forefoot/midfoot, and almost all contact closer to their body than they do in shoes. This is somewhat similar to the changes we observed in the posture review above. When the contact point, posture, and swing of the pendulum are tight together, things are more efficient. Contacting closer to the body means forces are applied much closer to the center of the joints. Very large decreases in the lever arm acting on the hip and knee have been observed (between 32–52 percent) when running barefoot. In a world where changes between *shoe A* and *shoe B* might amount to only 1–15 percent difference, these barefoot numbers are *very big* shifts. *Full disclosure:* As big as these numbers are, we don't know if this reduction is enough to prevent injury. However, it is clearly a move in the right direction.

	Overstride with heel landing	Pendulum-like stride (close to COM)	Overstride with forefoot landing
Effect on loading rate	Typically high (not because of heel landing, but because foot is far in front of COM)	Minimize	Typically lower than that of overstrided heel landing, but can still be high if landing too stiff
Effect on economy	Increased muscle work due to increased rise and fall of COM	Maximize elastic recoil	High metabolic cost to try to soften the landing (typically seen in runners with limited hip extension)

So putting all this information together shows that the barefoot running style with a forefoot contact is an effective method to decrease loading rate. However, it is not always the most efficient one. A neutral posture and a contact close to the center of mass appear to be very powerful factors to minimize loading rate *without a ding in metabolic cost*. In my professional experience with cueing gait and visualizing the corresponding changes in forces, I allow the foot contact style to be an effect, not a cause. That is, I cue the runner to maintain good posture and land closer to their center of mass at any given intensity. This preserves all the guidelines put forth above in the economy discussion. Whether someone defaults to a forefoot, midfoot, or rearfoot contact style is unique to their soft tissue mobility, speed, and limb length, but not my chief concern. Contact style is *not* the only way to decrease loading rate. It's possible to have lower loading rates with multiple foot contact styles by maintaining a neutral posture with good core control and by contacting close to your body.

So I Am Currently Pain-free. Should I Change My Running Form?

The first thing you should do is put better parts into your machine. Make sure you pass the "nonnegotiable three." If you don't, you are likely running suboptimally—maybe not from an injury standpoint, but from an efficiency

a   b   c

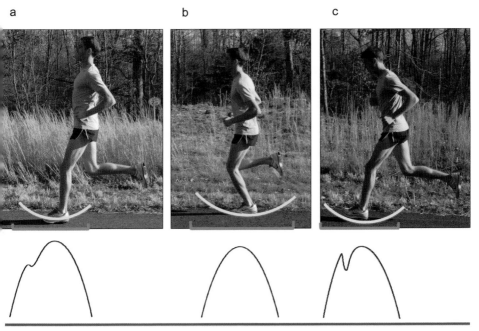

*The effect of a) backseat running, b) good alignment, and
c) toilet bowl syndrome on loading rates.*

ne. Improving your body will boost your running-form potential. Trying to
adjust form first is great to raise awareness, but don't be surprised if you fatigue
quickly and resort back to your old self because you don't yet have the control
you need. It's easy to make changes in your running form if your parts work
correctly. However, if the body is lacking, you need to stay consistent with *body
improvements* to allow *form improvements*. That's number one.

Now that we have got optimal parts, let's look back at the idea of "changing
form when nothing is wrong" from another angle. The research literature doesn't
point out any need to change form if things are going well. I do research, too,
but I'm first and foremost a clinician. There is a big difference between groups
of healthy runners and the "*n of 1*" patient who sits before me on the table. If
you have any history of patellofemoral joint pain, tibial stress syndrome, compartment syndrome, a prior tibial plateau stress fracture, or knee osteoarthritis,
applying forces at a great distance from the center of the joint is not smart.

One aim of this book is to get you to look beyond symptoms and try to
pinpoint the real cause of your imbalance. A gait style that allows you to land
too far in front of the body increases the lever arm and resulting loads on a
number of structures. Since we really can't decrease the peak GRF without a
huge ding in running economy, we need to move the force closer to the joint

center. Moving the foot contact "pendulum" closer in will minimize biomechanical wear and tear without impacting economy. Put more simply: Overstriding
will tremendously increase long-term complications for the above conditions.

So how do I do this? Is it all about foot strike?

It is true that the majority of runners will find themselves moving closer to
a midfoot landing if they pull their other factors in line (posture, landing close
to your body at a given speed, and using more glutes). However, I'm not a fan
of telling someone to land on a certain spot on your foot. Why? Landing on
the forefoot doesn't fix everything. Some barefoot runners land on the forefoot
in what we loosely call "bad barefoot" or what I call "fairy running" (basically a
forefoot style while overstriding). Their loading rate is really low, but there is
a huge metabolic cost to this and the lever arm acting on the knee is still quite
large. Think about the foot contact style as the effect and not the cause. When
trying to decrease lever arms and loading rate, it's where you land in relation to
your center of mass that counts.

The only reason to put the foot in front of the body when running is to store
elastic energy in the slingshot. It doesn't matter if it lands on the forefoot, the
midfoot, or the rearfoot; it just needs to land in the right spot. *The right spot* is
the place where the loading rate is the lowest and the metabolic cost of lower-
ing the body is down during contact. If you land too far in front of the center
of mass, your efficiency goes down and your loading rate goes up. High loading
rates are a very important causative factor for some but not all injuries. If you
have a limitation in getting the leg behind you (from a tight hip flexor, ankle, or
big toe) or have postural instability, you are likely going to land with a higher
loading rate. Don't stress. Just set aside time to improve your limiting factors.

Once the leg is directly under the center of mass, the maximum elastic energy is stored in the slingshot, and the body is under maximum load as the vertical forces are pushing down at their peak. To master this stage, you must have
excellent stability, not just at the spine, but in all planes of motion around all
the weight-bearing joints. If you can't generate a sufficient muscular response
to keep your parts stable during midstance, tissues become overwhelmed, and
injury ensues. Let's state our mantra yet one more time: High forces through
unstable levers is a recipe for disaster.

Finally, muscles hold taught as the slingshot is released and the body move
up and forward over a stable stance leg. The glutes capitalize on their leverage, and supply more of the force for push off as pace increases. Do you have
what it takes to do all of the above correctly? In Chapter 9, we'll take a look at
where your weak links are, and in Chapter 10 we'll upgrade your body.

The goal is to decrease the biomechanical loading on the body while minimizing energy cost, not raising it. If you can successfully lower your loading rates from the right method, you've found the Holy Grail of running form. It's nothing special or proprietary. It's all about using your body correctly, balancing out the force demands on the body. Balance is good. A lack of balance equals overload and a broken body . . . which brings us to our last point.

"I am in pain, is there anything I should do for my form?" Yes! Check out the gait cueing table for some very specific ways to address specific gait issues that cause pain in specific places. Shifting your form will help offset the strain on the injured area. While this is something for the short term for sure, there is nothing wrong with adopting any of these strategies long term. Let your body adapt!

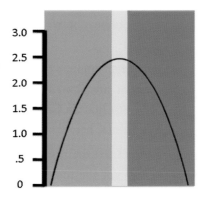 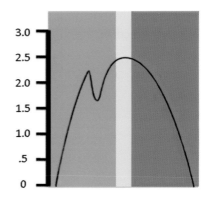

Is it the journey or the destination? Some tissues are injured when forces are too high (the destination), and others are injured when the force is applied too quickly (during the journey). Above, we have two graphs of the vertical GRF. On the left, we see a smooth rise in the slope of the curve. On the right, we see a steeper slope of the GRF. In both cases, the goal of the loading phase is to store energy. However, the steeper loading rate during this energy storage phase on the right creates problems for certain injuries such as stress fractures. Too high of a loading rate can overwhelm bone. If the injury heals but the gait mechanics are not fixed, there is a very high risk for repeat injury. This runner should receive cues to land close to his body, with a compliant limb, in good postural alignment so that his graph looks closer to that on the left side.

Other injuries are more attributed to the high forces that occur in midstance (the destination). Our mantra for this book has been high forces through unstable levers equals disaster. This force of 2.5x's body weight can overwhelm an unstable hip and allow increased rotational plane movement that is contributing to the runner's chronic IT band problems. In this case, the focus should be on improving the stabilization of the hip to meet the known demands that occur at midstance. Why can't we try to minimize the peak forces like we adjusted the loading rate? It is possible to raise or lower your peak force, but it requires severe compensations and is very inefficient. Instead of trying to lower the amount of force, time would be well spent improving the strength and stability of the hip stabilizers so they can rise to the occasion mile after mile.

Gait Fault	Problem	Why address the problem?	Correction
High Loading Rate	Loading structures too fast causes excessive wear and tear. High loading rates play a role in both stress fractures and soft tissue dysfunction.	Decreasing the loading rate applied to tissues will minimize tissue stress, minimizing the effects of the microtrauma of endurance training. Methods to decrease loading rate involve a combination of: a) encouraging a foot contact style closer to the body's center of mass, b) minimizing excessive lumbar arch (which shifts the body's center of mass backwards in relation to foot contact), c) changing limb stiffness.	*Take-home:* a. Simply "running softer" has been shown to decrease loading rates. b. Increasing cadence causes the foot to land closer to the body's structure and decreases energy absorbed into the body structure. Try to increase your cadence between 5-10% c. Correct lumbar alignment as mentioned in "Lower Quarter Crossed Syndrome" below. d. Heel-lift drill is a good cue to get the foot to land close to you and use your glute.
Increased Internal Hip Rotation	The incidence of PFPS and illiotibial band pain, and general anterior knee pain is typically associated with increases in peak internal hip rotation during stance.	The rotational alignment of the athlete hips should reflect your structural alignment. While some rotation of the hips (about 12-15 degrees) is a normal part of coupled motion, excessive mobility in the transverse plane creates mechanics for a number of lower extremity injuries.	*Take-home:* a. "Imagine the kneecaps as flashlights." Shine them forward as you run. b. On the treadmill, place a mirror in front of you to see what you are doing. If you see lots of rotation to the inside, try to keep it to a minimum as you run. Strengthen: get to work on lateral and hip extension strength.

Gait Fault	Problem	Why address the problem?	Correction
Quad-dominant Running Gait, i.e. tight hip flexors	To run a certain speed, you have to have a given stride length. Tight hip flexors prevent the pendulum from moving equally forward and backward around you. The path of the pendulum is shifted forward in space, making your foot contact excessively in front of the center of mass.	This increases compression of the patella in the trochlear groove and leads to increased muscle fatigue of the quads at a given intensity. Cueing the foot to land closer to the body minimizes the lever arm around the knee, which decreases shear stress on the knee. This is the most frequently seen cause of anterior knee pain in runners.	*Mobility:* Runners who are tight must increase hip extension through stretching hip flexors. See the mobility section of Ch. 10. *Drill to shift muscle memory:* Do 20-30 "chairs of death" squats before you go out for your run to cue your glute. *Change gait style:* Instead of driving the knee up and forward with the hip flexors, use the hamstring and glute to lift the heel up (as if doing a standing hamstring curl to 90 degrees).

Gait Fault	Problem	Why address the problem?	Correction
Lower Quarter Cross Syndrome, a.k.a. F.A.T.S.	While we somewhat jokingly called this F.A.T.S., this is a common pattern described by legendary physical therapist Dr. Janda. These postural patterns cause inhibition of the deep core muscles, glutes, hamstrings, and intrinsic foot muscles and an overactivation of the lumbar erectors, hip flexors, and calves.	The movement pattern dysfunction is not running specific, but this postural driven inhibition pattern transfers into the gait. To correct this pattern, you need to cue into lumbar neutral in standing, walking, drills, and running.	*Cue:* Keep the pelvis in neutral and dropping the sternum forward just enough so that the weight bias felt on the foot moves from the heel to the midfoot. Maintain this position as you run flat or uphill. To maintain lumbar neutral downhill, imagine a skier keeping their upper body perpendicular to the hill to avoid migration into lumbar extension.

Gait Fault	Problem	Why address the problem?	Correction
Wide or Narrow Base of Support	Excessive deviation from medial to lateral (or lateral to medial) imparts excess coronal plane forces that the runner is required to stabilize.	Often increased deviation in this plane is seen when the runner lacks adequate hip and core stability.	*To cue wider stance:* Run on a track or bike lane so that the second toe is on the edge of the line of the track. *To cue narrower stance:* Contact so that the foot lands in the center of the line as you run.
Medial Tibial Stress Syndrome	During stance, the muscles in the posterior medial compartment (inside of the shin) must slow the rate of pronation.	With a wider stance, the center of pressure is moved medial to the ankle joint center thus decreasing the demand of the muscles in the inside of the shin from being overworked.	*Cue:* Slightly widen the stance so that the second toe lands on the edge of the white line on track or bike lane. *Shoes:* A more minimally constructed shoe that doesn't stick out far from the foot also helps move the pressure more towards the inside of your foot. Make sure you strengthen the big toe!

Gait Fault	Problem	Why address the problem?	Correction
Achilles Tendinosis	While improving proper big toe and forefoot stability is paramount for this injury, these runners often exhibit a "positive ankle power" right at contact. Translation: At a time when you should be absorbing energy in the Achilles, you instead try to generate force.	Increasing concentric work (power generation) of the gastroc-soleus complex at contact causes a strain distribution problem in the Achilles that causes chronic imbalance. An unstable foot/ankle worsens situation by placing high loads through an unstable lever.	Medial/Lateral Stability: Emphasize contact of the triangle: medial and lateral ball of the foot, and the end of the big toe. Drill: Stand so that you face a wall two feet away. Keep your entire foot on the ground and allow your body to roll forward at the ankle so that you "fall" into the wall. Use your hands to stop chest from hitting the wall. The goal is to avoid the tendency to push off at the ankle and then replicate while running. When running, think about keeping the ankle loose.

Summary

- A strong stable runner with excellent core control can keep the spine in neutral running flat, uphill, or downhill. Imagine this stable core as the pivot point of the pendulum (your leg swinging back and forth beneath you). Check out the vertical compression test in Chapter 9 for more instruction on finding a neutral spine position.

- Full mobility of the hip, ankle, and ball of the foot ensures that the pendulum can swing equally in front and behind the center of mass. For a given speed, the person who contacts closer to their body is more efficient. A greater swing of the pendulum requires more force to swing the leg in front of and behind the body.
  - ✦ From contact to midstance—elastic energy is stored in the slingshot
  - ✦ From midstance to toe-off—energy is released through the slingshot
- If you have full mobility to get the leg behind you and you have excellent core control, the glute max will be able to perform its chief functions:
  - ✦ Postural: maintaining the upright position of the trunk
  - ✦ Propulsion: as speed increases, the hip supplies more and more of the propulsion force. Forceful hip extension is a critical component, as the glute max has the best mechanical leverage of any muscle in the body. Use it! When running correctly, you should feel as if you are "running from the butt."
- During midstance, your stability training comes into play as forces are highest. These forces peak with the increase of speed. It's critical that you have the control to minimize shifts or compensations in the lateral and rotational planes at the spine, hip, and foot. A stable body is one that can better use elastic energy.
- Don't overstride—imagine the pendulum moving equally in front and in back of you at all speeds. As speed increases, so must your stride length. But this increased "arc of the pendulum" needs to increase equally on both sides and not just out in front.
  - ✦ The heel lift drill can improve focus for using more muscles on the back side of the leg and less on the front side of the leg. Using more muscles, with each doing less work, is more mechanically efficient and provides more resistance to fatigue.
- On downhills, avoid the temptation to lean back and put on the brakes. Instead, lean ever so slightly forward, almost like you are "skiing" down the hill. Train to increase your cadence so your feet can stay closer to you.

- On uphills, a natural forward lean into the hill is helpful to decrease the lever arm on the contact leg. However, taking faster, shorter steps on steeper hills ease the work your muscles do for each step.
- Good stability plus good posture plus good pendulum plus optimal stance time equal maximizing recoil.
- There is no single best strategy for running form for everyone, but if you can minimize the loading rate (better for tissue strain), while maximizing the elastic recoil, you have found the Holy Grail.

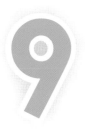

Assessment and Development of the Athlete Within— Redefining the Body You've Come to Know and Love

Remember the Nike ad, "*Be like Mike*" (Jordan)? Remember all that nice inspirational stuff we had in Chapter 1 encouraging you to find your inner athlete? So far we've given you lots of information to think about how and why your body has gotten to where it is now. You know this "mold" you've created for your body over the years? It's time to smash it into a billion little pieces and start working on the *You 2.0.*

Every coach out there worth his weight establishes some type of *performance plan* for your "engine." You can find out what your fitness level is by using recent race splits or time trials. They provide reference points on your cardiovascular adaptations and fitness. Based on this information, you can set long-term goals as well as smaller ones to keep you focused and on track. As new milestones are reached, your training intensity should also increase to ensure that you are progressing towards your end goal. The key is to stay on top of your game. While this is a great way to determine the type of physiologic stress you need in training, it completely ignores the biomechanical factors that affect you as a runner.

If you still aren't seeing the value in thinking outside F.I.T., let me present the following. Let's pretend you are a coach (if you aren't already).

Stats show that 82 percent of runners will get injured. This means that 82 percent of runners *you are responsible for* will get injured. If you are lucky, this occurs sometime in the off-season. If you aren't lucky, it occurs one week before the district/state/national meet and you lose your top-scoring runner. Wish you had taken some time to look outside the box when you had the chance? Would a better understanding of the previous chapters' of techno-babble have changed the way you dealt with your runners' aches and pains? Do you wish you could find out the specifics of each runner's chassis adaptations to ensure they can successfully apply their newfound horsepower and reduce their injury risk?

Remember Laird's quote, "Train for what you don't know"? We can't forecast every challenge facing every one of us, but we can know more by looking for answers. In my day job, I collect objective data on each and every runner who walks in the door. Honestly, an assessment in my lab is like cheating. It tells me exactly where the imbalances are in a runner's gait, when they occur, and exactly how much. It shows me exactly *what* types of mechanical stress affect the runner while running. While this information is critical to the level of biomechanical assessment I provide, it's useless without a thorough understanding of *why* the runner moves the way he does. To understand this, you need to look at his individual limitations and strengths in both mobility and stability. So sure, compensations in your running form can adversely affect tissue load, but more typically, deficits in mobility and strength will cause compensations in your running form.

Mobility and stability deficits are the driving factors behind tissue overload that cause typical overuse injuries in running. When you get hurt, it's easy to narrow your focus to the location of pain and block everything else out. However, this is not the smartest move if you really want to fix the problem. For most running injuries, *the causative mechanics behind different injuries are rather similar*. Still not clear enough? Think about this: You may have chronic shin pain that is really the result of poor foot control. However, poor foot control could just as easily cause you to have a metatarsalgia, Achilles tendinopathy, plantar fasciitis, sesmoiditis, compartment syndrome, or even stress fractures. So if you fix the factors driving your problem, you not only help your current problem, you also decrease your chances of getting another injury related to the same cause. Imbalances that take our body away from the norm cause problems, and these problems are usually present well before you have pain. Don't get hurt or let your athletes get hurt on your watch. Get rid of the weak links, build a better athlete, and bring better ingredients to the table.

So Exactly What Does a Runner Need to "Bring to the Table"?

If you really are seeking to improve your performance and send running njuries walking the other direction, your body needs to be able to run as a nobile, strong, and stable spring. To do this, you need to have certain physical ttributes that are nonnegotiable (yes, you've seen this before, and yes, it's *that* mportant):

1. Enough mobility to get the leg behind you in stance.
2. Stability of the core, hips, and foot to maintain posture and optimize transfer of energy.
3. Strength and power from the glute to drive the body up and forward.

This is a very specific list that unites all of our conceptual understanding hus far. But it's still abstract. How do you define "enough"? You don't guess; ou establish specific tests to identify what your unique needs are as a runner.

What follows is a summary of each test, why it is important, and what you an do to improve. The tests are based on objective criteria to define limita-ions in your tissue length and mobility, and to uncover neuromuscular coor-lination deficits, muscle dominance patterns, and strength limitations. The nobility tests are all very specific so that one test looks for one variable. The tability tests have a bit of overlap. Why? People use different control strategies o move their slightly different parts. Looking at things from more than one pecific angle gives more perspective on the way someone moves.

Mobility Tests	Stability Tests
Ankle dorsiflexion	Vertical compression posture
Big toe dorsiflexion	Bridge
Hip flexor mobility	Bilateral squat
Hamstring	Big toe stabilization
Tissue flossing	Single-leg squat

Recently, lots of screening tests have come out that aim to identify limitations in our athletes. One of these is the Functional Movement Screen (FMS). The FMS is a very good way to *generally* assess *general* limitations that *generally* affect someone. That's a lot of "generals"! Let's say someone received a certain subpar score on the FMS. That score doesn't really point out the *specific* issue with that person. Even with all my years of musculoskeletal experience, if the runner failed a part of the FMS, I'd still need to dig deeper to identify their *specific* problem. So instead of looking at generalities, let's look at the specifics.

When Is the Best Time to Take the Tests?

Now! While I wouldn't say it's smart to go through this testing sequence if you are 100 percent spent from an intense workout that day or the day prior, there is no reason to taper for these tests. You'd like to see what you can learn from yourself under normal circumstances. If you are training, normal circumstances likely means that you get tired and fatigued on some days and feel better on other days.

Can I Do These Tests If I'm Injured?

Do as much as you can. Some runners' perspective is that they don't want to test if they are resting or just coming back from time off. I think we've made a pretty clear case that rest doesn't *improve* tissues. The earlier you get to work on your issues, the sooner you'll improve them.

Benched for the season? OK, so your nightmare came true. You have an injury that is severe enough that your MD/PT cut you off from running for a while. Maybe you are even in a boot or on crutches. Going to reduced weight bearing and no running for weeks on end is a total bummer, I know. Does this mean you should just stick to the pool running and minimize your losses? My inability to sit still has made me the king of rehab. There are a dozen exercises in this book that require no weight bearing on the lower leg at all. If you plan right, you can even *improve* some of your limitations at other joints during this time. As soon as you find out what you *can't* do, think about what you *can* do, and get to work!

What If I Fail a Test?

Failing any one of these tests doesn't mean you are a poor runner. It doesn't mean you aren't trying, and it doesn't mean you are going to get injured tomorrow. For example: While I can't say that every runner with limited hip extension has poor running economy, I can say that about 99 percent of runners I've tested with poor running economy have decreased hip extension. This assessment is tailored to isolate variables that are roadblocks to your performance potential and injury risk. I love the following quote from *Evolution in Four Dimensions* by Eva Jablonka and Marion J. Lamb: "If you are advising or treating individuals according to the average effects, you may be doing the wrong thing." Everyone doing the same stuff isn't the best use of your time. Everyone has a different weak link in their chain. Finding your link and getting directional guidance on how to fix it helps develop you as a well-rounded athlete.

How Do I Use This Screening Tool?

Read through the detailed test descriptions that follow. It always helps to know why you are doing something. While it's possible to do these solo, it's a bit easier to grab a partner. Check out the table at the end of this chapter. It contains the name of each test, what the critical aspect of each test is, and exactly what to focus on to improve your deficits. Record your results for now to keep all this info straight in your head and for reference later so you can see your improvement. If you pass, congratulations. If you fail, now is not the time for tears. Simply follow the plan to correct the problems found. All of the corrective exercises are listed in the next chapter. The exercises that follow to improve mobility (both tissue length and glide) are color coded blue. OK, it's go time!

Disclaimer

This algorithm is a highly effective tool, as the imbalances we measure in a runner's form are typically revealed in their musculoskeletal exam. Ever heard the saying, "Don't look for the one zebra in a field of horses"? People can compensate a thousand different ways for a certain weakness or mobility limitation, and you'll always find a zebra that doesn't quite fit the mold. If something is confusing during your own self-assessment, or when assessing one of your athletes or patients, find someone who is one pay grade higher to help you out. You'll often find that talking it out helps make things clearer. And if you are still stumped, go see a professional—a physical therapist or physician who specializes in treating runners. A major goal of this book is to give you information to help you help yourself. In the front there is the nice legal disclaimer that says that none of the information in this book is designed to diagnose your condition and that you should seek medical help when you deem appropriate. If you are stumped, or things aren't progressing as you'd expect, know when to call in the expert. A formal evaluation from a trusted health professional is still the *most specific* way to make sure you are taking the right course of action. After several hundred pages, you should be able to help the horses. Leave the zebras to folks trained to deal with them.

Mobility Assessments

Test 1: Dorsiflexion of ankle

Sit down on a chair so that your knee and ankle are both bent at 90 degrees. Keeping your foot in the exact same place on the ground, slide your hips forward so that the front of your knee is just past your toes. If you can't keep your heel on the ground in this position, your Achilles is too tight.

Proper flexibility of the Achilles is necessary to allow the foot to get behind the hips for effective toe-off. Without this flexibility, you'll overstress the area in lower-heeled minimal shoes, and, more importantly, change the way you store and release elastic energy, which compromises effective push-off.

How to improve:

- **Do a burrito Achilles/calf stretch.** This is the good, old-fashioned runner's calf stretch with a twist. First, fold a hand towel into a burrito. Place this towel roll under your big toe only, with the outside of your foot on the ground—this "locks out" the foot, making sure that you actually lengthen the Achilles and don't just pronate the foot as you lean into the wall. With that leg slightly behind the body, lean into the wall, keeping the heel on the ground. Hold for three minutes on each side. (Yes, three minutes is how long research shows we need to hold stretches for tissues that are too short.) It can take 10–12 weeks to improve soft tissue length. If you are seeking faster gains, check out the soleus and "calf smash" soft tissue release techniques in Chapter 10. Yes, tissue mobilization is quite aggressive, but it is highly effective for improving tissue glide and much quicker than stretching alone.

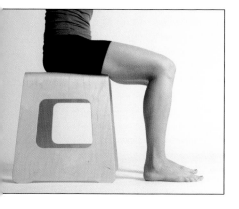
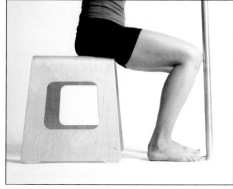

Test 2: Dorsiflexion of big toe

Keeping your body in the same position as the end of Test 1, reach down and grab your big toe. While keeping the ball of the foot flat on the ground, raise the big toe up (keeping it straight) until it is 30 degrees above the ground. If you can't raise it to 30 degrees, or if you find that the ball of your foot comes off the floor while trying to raise it, your plantar fascia is too tight.

Proper range here allows you to roll straight through the ball of the foot at toe-off. If tight, efficiency is compromised since your push-off is cut short. Additionally, if you can't roll straight through the forefoot, your foot will either spin inward or outward, and this can decrease support from the all-important big toe outward, and this leads to injuries farther up the leg.

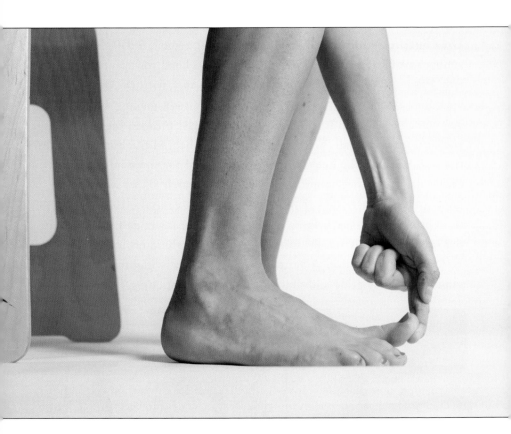

How to improve:

- **Improve plantar fascia mobility.** The plantar fascia is an extremely dense, tight tissue that doesn't respond well to stretching. It's better to think about breaking up tight spots within the plantar fascia to improve its mobility. This approach produces changes faster than stretching and is much more specific.

  Sit down and cross one leg over another with your top ankle on your knee. Press your thumbs firmly into the bottom of the foot. The plantar fascia runs like a triangle from the heel to the ball of the foot. Poke around for areas that feel sore. These sore places are overly restricted and bound down. Apply firm pressure and flex the toes back and forth to mobilize the area. Do this four to five minutes a day for about three weeks or until soreness alleviates.

Test 3: Hip extension

Kneel down on one knee, inside a door jamb, such that the femur of the leg you are kneeling on is vertical and the tibia of the opposite leg is vertical. In the picture, a vertical bar was used instead of the doorway to provide a better visual, but it's the exact same idea. In this position, you'll naturally have a bit of space between your lower back and the wall. Tilt your pelvis backwards so that the hollow between your lower back and the doorjam disappears (imagine tilting a bowl of cereal so that it spills behind you). Do you feel a stretch in the front of your thigh? If the answer is no, you likely have all the hip extension mobility you need to run. If the answer is yes, let's talk.

As running speed increases, more and more force needs to be generated from the hip. If you lack hip extension, you lose efficiency since the free elastic energy stored in the tendon can't move behind the body for full hip drive. Without the ability to extend the hip, the foot contacts further and further in front of the body as speed and stride length increases. Contacting too far in front of the body is associated with increased braking and vertical forces (critical for economy) and high loading rates (critical for injury risk). Further, limi-

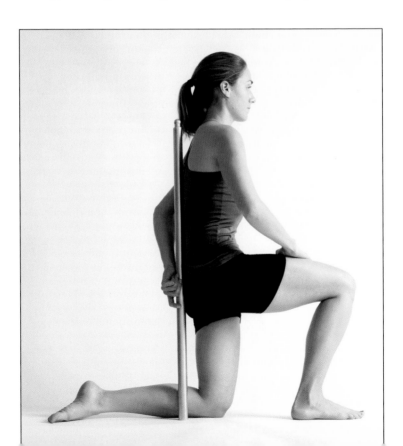

tations in hip extension compromise posture by forcing increased arch in the low back. These postural compensations directly impair core stability during running. Limitations in hip extension mobility on one side increase tension on the contralateral hamstring and are an often overlooked source of chronic hamstring strains. In short, you get a lot of problems due to one problem.

How to improve:

- Hip extension tightness is the most frequently seen problem in runners. Fortunately, it's very easy to remedy. Since this is ultimately a length issue, we'll attack it from two sides. The kneeling hip flexor stretch is a great way to open up the range of your psoas. Hold this position for 3–5 minutes daily. Think you can't find the time? Try to do your e-mail in this position. This stretch can be supercharged by using a rubber band to increase the load and help open up the capsule on the front of the hip. If you want to work on soft tissue mobility, check out the LAX ball section to mobilize the bound-up layers in your body.

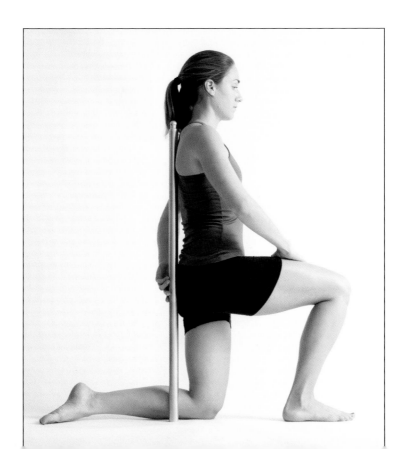

Test 4: Hamstring

Lie on your back with one leg straight out on the floor. Flex the other leg up so you can interlace your fingers behind the back of your thigh. Straighten your knee and pull the leg up to the ceiling. For distance runners, with the knee straight, you should be able to get the leg up to about 70 degrees of hip flexion. For steeplers and hurdlers, this angle needs to go past vertical to about 100 degrees, since taking the lead leg out to 95–100 degrees of hip flexion is a requirement that other distance runners don't have. At these end limits, it's OK to feel a mild stretch in the back of the leg. However, if you feel death-grip tightness in the back of the leg, it obviously means that things are too tight and could use some extra motion.

The big conspiracy theory is that everyone has tight hamstrings. Most folks think that you need 90 degrees to run, and you really don't (again, unless you need more motion due to running a steeple of hurdles). But you never know until you check, right? Hamstring tightness limits the motion of your pelvis on your hip causing compensatory roundness of the low back and loss of core stabilization. They are also a contributing factor to hamstring strains.

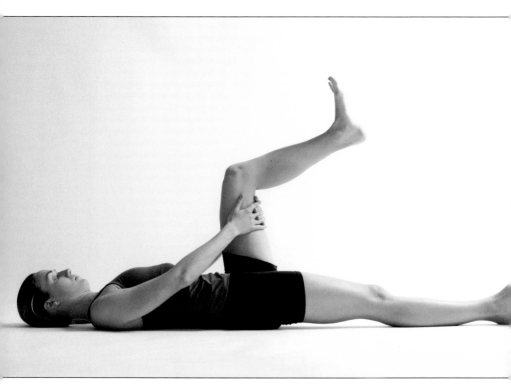

How to improve:

- The test position becomes the stretch, although using a doorway is a nice option to hold the leg up since you'll be there for 3–5 minutes. Want other options? Grab the LAX ball and check out the tissue mobility work in the treatment session. One word of caution: If you feel any sharp electrical or "zingy" sensations when doing this stretch, call your clinician of choice. This test is also a way to identify problems with nerves, tension, and compression. Nerves don't like to be stretched, and doing so will actually make them worse.

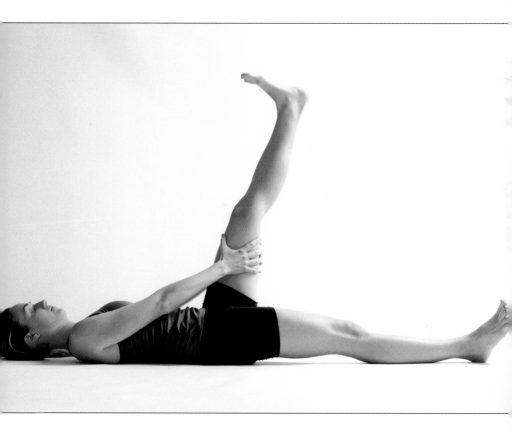

Test 5: Tissue flossing

The repetitive aspect of running places compound stresses on the body. Just as the body tries to recover from a previous workout, additional load is applied through today's workout. The body will first and foremost make attempts to keep itself intact; however, it needs some help in keeping tissues supple throughout the remodeling process. The act of mobilizing scar tissue to keep the normal shortening and lengthening of connective tissues intact is termed "tissue flossing." A lot of runners have exposure to this concept with the foam roller. However, there are many other tissues in the body that need freeing up which we neglect. Let's change that.

Truth be told, this really isn't so much of a specific pass/ fail. Rather, it's more about you establishing an ongoing relationship with your body. Your body belongs to you. Don't be afraid to poke around and see if you find things you don't like. When you find areas of excessive adhesion, it's up to you to work them out. In the end, this leads to a better recovery. Check out the guided tour in the mobility section.

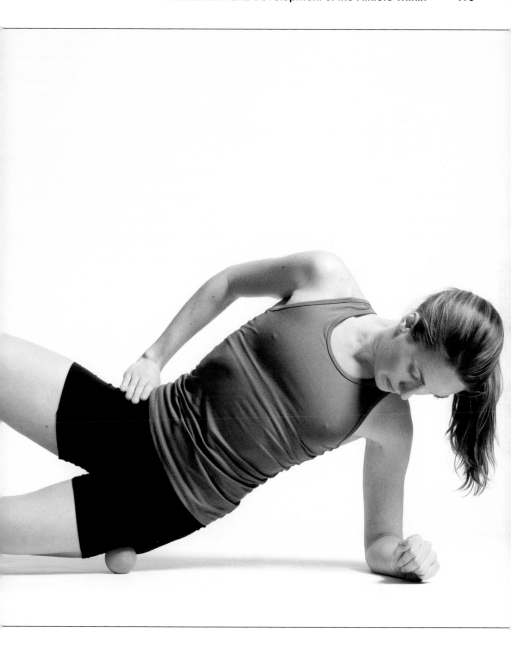

Test 6: Vertical compression test for postural alignment

This test can be done solo, but having a partner can help greatly. Stand with your feet in a comfortable width. First, think about where your weight is. More in the heels? Evenly distributed throughout the entire foot? Your partner should stand behind you with their hands on your shoulders. While you are relaxed (not overly tensing the abdominals), your partner should press down firmly on your shoulders. What happens to your posture? Does their downward pressure cause your spine to buckle and move into a more arched position, or do you stand firm with weight evenly distributed through the entire foot?

Most runners have a tendency to stand, walk, and thus, run in the "backseat." Since this slumped posture feels normal, it is adopted in their running form. Unfortunately, this posture significantly decreases your ability to use your core strength, shifts your center of mass back, and causes you to land too far in front of the center of the body. It accentuates your overstride.

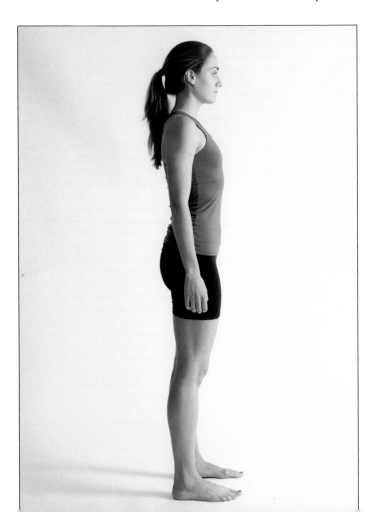

Further, this postural fault makes it tough for you to activate the hip foot stabilizers. All of these effects make you more prone to fatigue and form changes when running. If you need to improve the way your parts work, step one is to put them in a better position.

• **Fixing your posture**. To use the forefoot for balance, you first need to have weight equally distributed over your forefoot and rearfoot. To find the correct position, place one hand on your belly button and one hand on your sternum. Imagine that the hand on your bellybutton is blocking your pelvis from shifting forward. Then drop the upper hand and sternum forward slightly so that you have a slight bend at the waist (not the ankle and knee) until you feel weight equally distributed over the forefoot and rearfoot. Make this your new normal posture. The more you practice good posture when not running, the easier it will be to find and maintain it mile after mile.

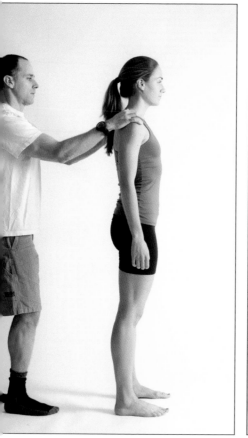
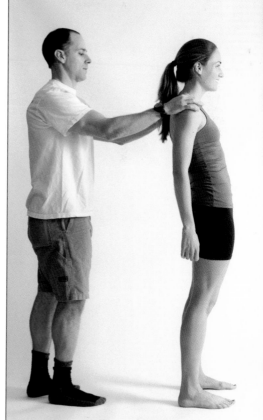

Test 7: Bilateral squat

Either have a friend watch you from the side or film yourself. Step into the viewfinder at a right angle to the camera. You are looking for a profile shot, not of your face but of your muscle mechanics. Place hands on hips, complete five squats, and then replay your movie. We are looking for dominance of the quads or dominance of the glutes. When you come down, your lower leg (tibia) should be able to remain completely vertical. You should look like you are sitting down in a chair behind you. If you notice that your knees and lower leg move forward in each squat, we need to discuss how your bad habits and movement skills will creep into your gait.

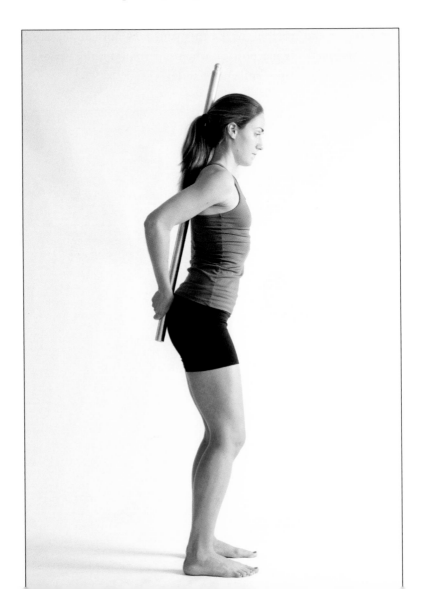

One of the critical aspects we discussed in the gait chapter is adopting a foot contact "pendulum" that keeps the leg swing even on both sides of the body. Runners who initiate their squat by bringing the hips backwards better utilize their hip extension, contact closer to their body, and thus run more efficiently. However, if you initiate your squat by moving the knees forward, you are much more likely to stride out in front of the body when running. This pattern is responsible for increasing the lever arm (and thus load) to the knee and is a limiter of efficiency.

- **Fixing muscle imbalances.** Changing from a quad-dominant strategy to a glute dominant strategy can seem quite foreign. The "chair of death" is a very functional way to change your habits and force your glute to support and stabilize your body. This movement pattern training can be further complemented by both Phase 1 and Phase 2 hip stabilization exercises.

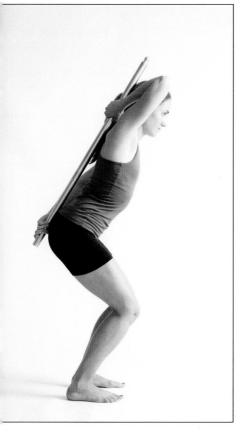
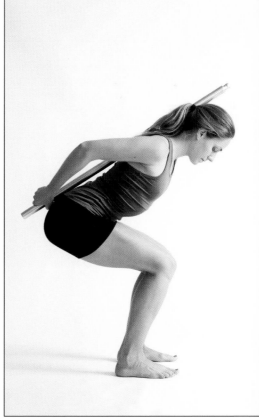

Test 8: Bridge

Lie on your back with knees bent and feet flat on the floor. Clasp your hands together and raise them up towards the sky. Now lift the hips off of the ground and hold for 30 seconds. Ask yourself which muscles you feel working. Next, raise one leg just a few inches off the floor. Hold for 30 seconds. Lower the leg down. Repeat on opposite side.

The goal of this test is to identify your "go to" muscles that move your hip. The glute max has two jobs: it moves your hip behind you into extension, and it also stabilizes you from a postural standpoint. So if you felt your glute doing all the work when you raised your butt off the floor on both legs then you are on the right track. But what if that is not what you felt, and what if your pelvis shifted or dropped as you lifted one leg?

If you said your lower back had any tightness, this is a big red flag. Tightness in the low back means you are trying to arch this back first and then move. This default pattern results in postural breakdown and needs to be rewritten. Correct running posture comes from extending the hip while keeping the spine stable. When raising one leg off the floor, you should be able to keep your pelvis stable enough to balance a full glass of red wine on your belly button while doing this test over Mom's brand new white carpet. The glute max should be providing the effort to both stabilize and lift the pelvis up. If you notice a drop in one side of your pelvis, a shift in the pelvis, or an overactive or "crampy" hamstring then you need to improve hip stability before you try to move it.

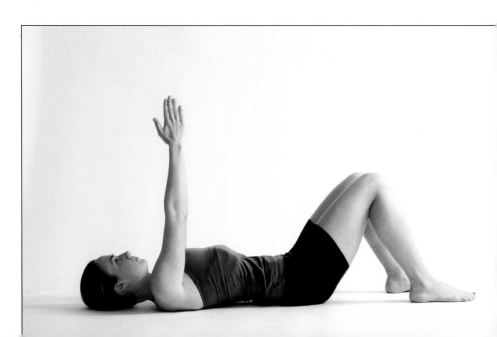

• **Triggering a broken butt.** Most runners who fail the vertical posture compression test and the hip extension test not only have a weak glute max, they also have a tough time even thinking about trying to turn it on. Instead of progressing to advanced exercises, it's best to take this in steps. Master the Stage 1 hip exercises first, and then progress onto the Stage 2 goods when you are ready.

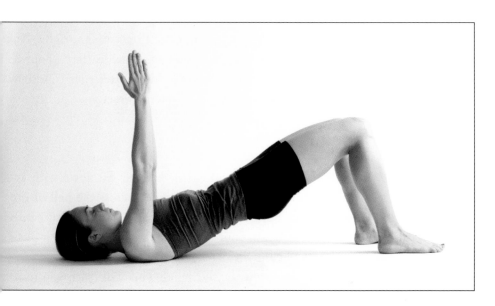

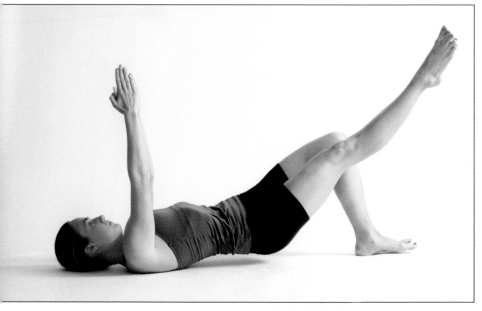

Test 9: Isolating the big toe

Standing, drive the big toe into the ground (plantar flexion) while slightly elevating the lesser toes (dorsiflexing). Make sure not to roll the ankle in or out to compensate. If you find that you tend to bend the joint in the big toe so that your toe curls, it's a sign that you are dominating with muscles up in the shin and not able to isolate specific muscles inside the foot.

The ability to isolate and coordinate movements of the big toe is what provides the specific control we need from the foot during the stance phase. Try to hammer a nail gripping it with only your four fingers. Pretty tough, right? Now wrap your thumb around the hammer and keep nailing. Much easier! About 85 percent of your foot control comes from the big toe. The better your coordination of muscles inside the foot, the faster you can microcorrect your position in stance.

How to improve:

- Learn to isolate the muscles controlling the big toe: Sit down with your foot flat on the floor with equal pressure applied across the ball of the foot. Place a thin book, a piece of hard plastic or a stiff piece of cardboard under the big toe. With your hand, tilt the board up. Then push straight down into the board with your big toe, keeping it straight, as you slowly resist this motion with your hand. This will teach you to isolate the big toe from the little toes. When you can do this, the test becomes the exercise.

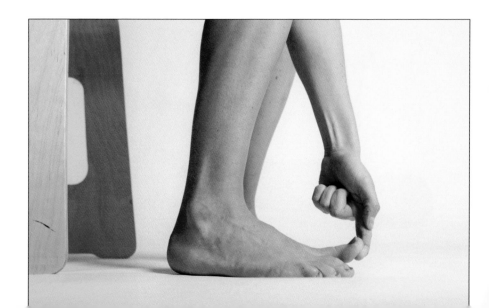

- Do "toe yoga." Simply try to raise/lower the little toes and big toe independently of each other to improve coordination. Do this several times a day until easily mastered. Since it's targeting a change in control and not strength, improvements are rapid—usually noticeable in a few days to two weeks.

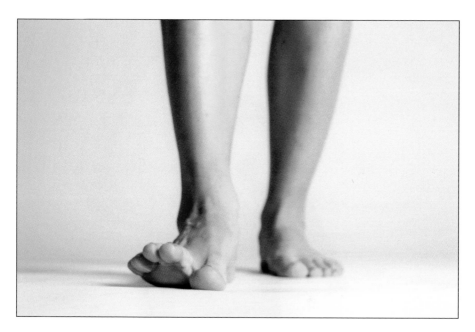

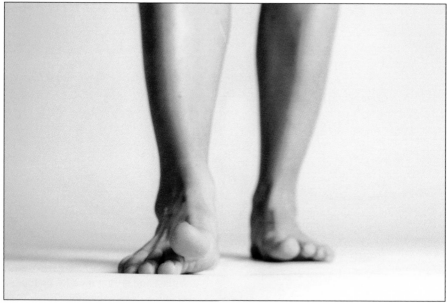

Test 10: Single-leg squat

Stand in front of your partner or video camera. You will perform six single-leg squats on each leg and score your performance to identify your limiters. Everyone starts out with a high score of 6/6 points. You'll lose a point for each issue we find according to the table on page 206.

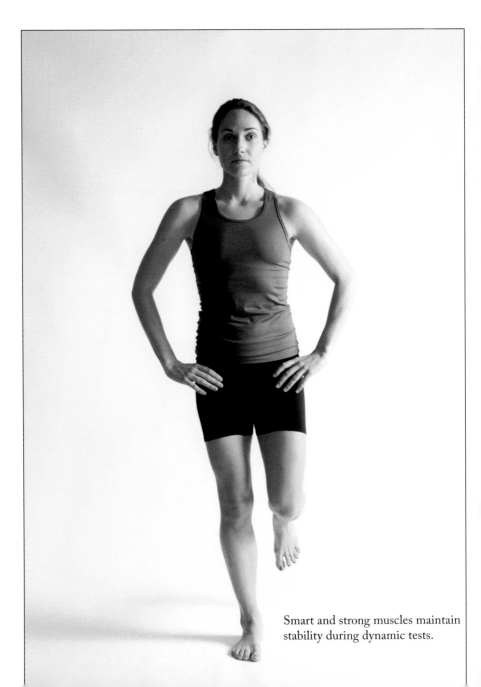

Smart and strong muscles maintain stability during dynamic tests.

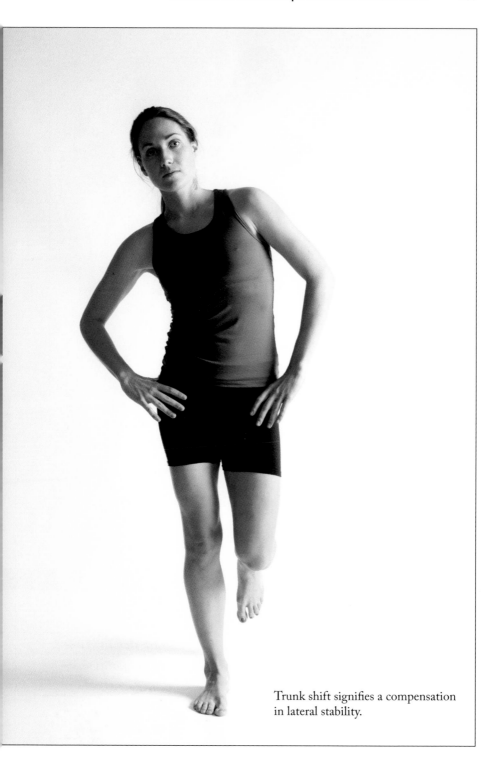

Trunk shift signifies a compensation in lateral stability.

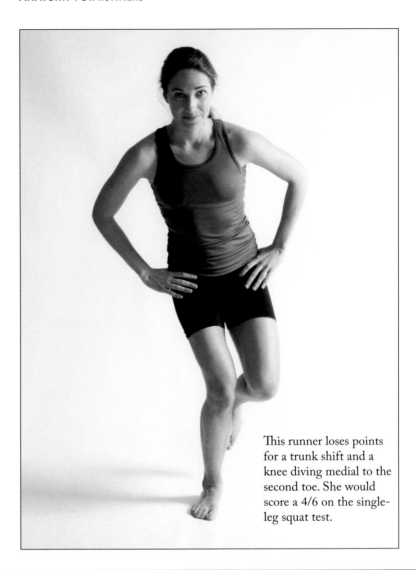

This runner loses points for a trunk shift and a knee diving medial to the second toe. She would score a 4/6 on the single-leg squat test.

Deductions	Scored Criteria	Implications
-1	Loss of foot contact	*Foot stability issue*
-1	Trunk shift	*Could be hip or foot issue*
-1	Pelvic drop	*Hip stability issue*
-1	Knee dives medial to second toe	*Hip stability issue*
-1	Hands come off hips	*Gross instability*
-1	Loss of balance	*Gross instability*
TOTAL: X/6		

Running is basically a bunch of single-leg squats with a flight phase in between. To run well, it's your responsibility to bring a stable body to the game. Just as you can't fire a cannon from a canoe, you can't push off from a bunch of unstable levers. Screening single-leg balance and squat reveals deficits that tell a lot about you as a runner. Problems here may show up immediately in your form or may mean you fatigue rapidly. What should we see?

Do you see someone who appears stable and solid or a wobbly mess? The body should not rock or wobble excessively when running, so why should it when performing tests and improving movement skills? Trunk shifts are usually in response to profound weaknesses in the lower body. The arms and trunk should be still and quiet so that stability is coming from the ankle and hip. If you see excessive wobbling in the foot (the inside ball of the foot and big toe repeatedly come off the ground), you have foot and ankle issues. If you see excessive leaning or shifting of the trunk, you likely have hip issues or you could be compensating for your foot. What is the difference? If your foot is stable and you are wobbling up top, it is likely just hip stability deficits. And if both look unsteady? It is likely both need tune-ups. The knee (the middle child) is stuck in the middle and does what it's told to do by the hip and the foot.

- Put more stability in a single-leg stance. You can view this as a top-down or bottom-up approach, but either way the body needs to work together. While good posture puts the pelvis into neutral for hip stabilization, it is also moves the center of body weight to the middle of the foot so that the big toe can do its job. We begin with good alignment, and then work into more complex movement skills to generate high forces like those during running. Check out the chart for ways to progress both the Phase 1 and Phase 2 stability programs. The ultimate goal is to improve your stability, strength, and skill to the point where running is not stressful to muscles that control the lateral and rotational planes.

Exercises focusing on making muscles *smarter* are purple, *stronger* are red, and *spring* (power) are green. Exercises focusing on tissue mobility are blue.

Test	Pass	Fail	Phase 1 Focus	Phase 2 Focus
Dorsiflexion of ankle		Stiffness in front of ankle	See your MD/PT	Continue until resolved
		Tightness in back	Stretch Achilles, soleus STW/calf smash	
Dorsiflexion of big toe		Pain on top of toe	See your MD/PT	Continue until resolved
		Tight/limited mobility	STW on plantar fascia	
Hip extension		Can't get back flat against doorframe without stretch in front of hip flexors	Kneeling hip flexor stretch, add band for deeper stretch, LAX ball in hip mobilization	Continue until resolved
Hamstring		Can't reach 70 degrees at hip	Hamstring STW/ stretching	Continue until resolved
Tissue flossing		Limited mobility or pain discovered through self-assessment	STW to alleviate trigger points	Ongoing throughout season

Test	Pass	Fail	Phase 1 Focus	Phase 2 Focus
Vertical compression test for postural alignment		Increase in lumbar lordosis with applied downward force	Postural practice all day, every day, single-leg balance	Single-leg balance with eyes closed, ball toss, Swiss ball torso rotation, Swiss ball Russian twist
Bilateral squat		Knees move forward when moving into squat	Chair of death, squat training	Rocker board squats, twisting lunges
Bridge		Feel low back tighten	Pigeon hip extension, Knee to chest, bridge, donkey kick	T-ball rock 'n' roll, single-leg dead lift, Swiss ball triad (unilateral)
		Pelvic drop/ rotation/shift	Clamshell, donkey kick, hip hike	Lateral hip bridge, rotisserie chicken, rotational lunge
Isolating the big toe		Can't drive big toe down without curling	Big toe isolation, toe yoga	Single-leg rocker board, single-leg balance with med ball throw

Test	Pass	Fail	Phase 1 Focus	Phase 2 Focus
Single-leg squat		Lose forefoot contact	Big toe/toe yoga/ balance	Rocker board, med ball throws in single-leg
		Trunk shift	If due to loss of foot contact, emphasize foot, if due to hip instability, emphasize hip	Same
		Knee dive inside second toe	Clamshells, hip hike	Single-leg deadlift, side hip abduction, rotisserie chicken
		Pelvic drop	Clamshells, hip hike	Side hip abduction, twisting lunge, Swiss ball rotations
		Loss of balance	Single-leg balance	Single-leg dead lift
		Hands off hips	Swiss ball rock 'n' roll	Russian twist

10

Putting Humpty Dumpty Back Together Again — Corrective Exercises

So you've done your screening. Your limitations are out there front and center. Isn't it great to know exactly what you have to work on? Throughout this book we've broken down every aspect of your anatomy and your running form. It's time to refine the parts and tune up the system.

As mentioned in Chapter 9, the following corrective exercises are grouped by their intended purpose.

Mobility—Purpose is to increase either tissue length or glide as needed for running.

- Length changes require stretching with long static holds of 3–5 minutes, 4–6 days a week, for about 10–12 weeks before the tissue adapts. Yes, this is a long time. Better start now, right? Periodically check your assessment and examine improvements. Once you've gotten full range, there is no need to continue.
- Tissue glide changes respond well to 3–5 minutes per body part. This can be done 3–7 days a week. You should notice significant improvements in tissue glide as you free up the sticky areas. If these spots are not improving, it means that the tissue strain is

still high, which is likely a stability problem. Doing self-assessments on tissue glide 1–2 times a week ensures that you keep tissues supple as you train.

- Eccentrics—lengthening contractions provide a stimulus to improve tendon strength. Since this occurs by reorganizing the tissues from "scattered straws" back to "straws aligned in a box" (see chapter on tissue mobility), it has merit as part of a tissue mobility approach and is listed here. Dosage of eccentrics is 40–60 reps. Mild/moderate pain during this exercise is OK.

Stability Training—Improve the control and power delivery of the musculoskeletal system to stabilize and propel the runner.

Put the most stable runner you can be into your running form. The more strategies you have, the closer you'll operate at your peak performance. This is broken up in the context of the strength chapter: *develop a smarter and stronger spring.*

- Stability needs to be built from the bottom up. While you may be able to get away with some advanced exercises, you'll likely do them wrong with lots of muscle substitutions. Changing your muscle memory is all about making the muscles *"smarter."* To train smart movements, you need to do 4,000–6,000 reps to change your body's perception of what feels normal. It is best to do them frequently throughout the day and 1–2 weeks initially to lay a foundation, as skimping on form here will produce big problems later. *Smarter* exercises improve coordination and cue specific muscles to work in the right way with correct postural alignment. While they won't set any records on muscle intensity, they likely will set records for you on brain intensity as you focus on form.
- Stronger: After you've learned the difference between moving right and wrong, then we can bump your efforts up with more advanced training. This means taking your smarter muscles into multiplane, full movemen activities with resistance to increase force generation by the body. The goal here is to make tissues *stronger.* Optimal doses for improvement

are 2–4 days a week. For maintenance, 1–2 days a week is all that is required.

- Spring: A big spring is stiff and capable of delivering incredible force in a short period of time. A big spring can directly improve elastic energy transfer within the body as well as your economy. The road to success here comes from intense heavy lifting, plyometrics. The volume of this type of effort is low, but the quality is 100 percent. These high force requirements mean you need to earn the right to train this way. If not, you won't obtain the benefits, and worse, might wind up injured. Olympic lifting instruction was purposely left out of this book. The technique is so critical that hands-on teaching sessions are required. Many successful strength coaches have their runners practice the technique of Olympic lifts for weeks to months before adding any weight at all. When you are ready to progress to this point, seek out some local help in your area.

Seriously? You want me to *add* something to my training plan?

"But wait . . . I'm busy. I'm in school and I have finals/work and I have a project due/ I'm a homemaker and I have a kid puking on me and another I have to pick up from soccer practice . . . and I need to get my run in or I'll go crazy! I don't have time!" Right? OK, if you don't want to make time, that's fine. Just don't expect any of this to improve. Imagine you are back in school and you are doing really well in civics but failing algebra. Studying harder in civics won't do a thing to raise your grade in algebra.

Simply adding or reducing running volume, or even resting, doesn't fix your biomechanical limitations as a runner. If any of you ever think you have all the stability you need, you should probably spend some time working on your ego as well. Great athletes don't *rest* with who they are. They *push* toward who they could be.

Tissue Mobility

You have to have enough mobility to run. Supple tissues work better, plain and simple. The following will keep you on track:

1. **Hamstring**—Sit on a LAX ball on tight spots within the hamstring. While leaning the majority of the body weight on the LAX ball, flex and extend your knee.

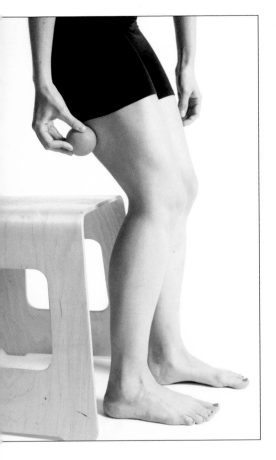 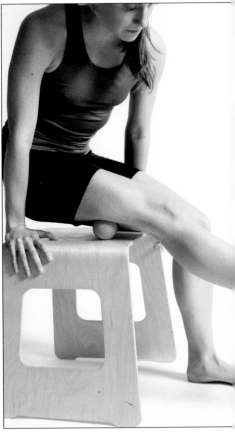

2. **Plantar fascia**—Apply pressure and flex and extend toes to open tissue tightness. Do this 3–5 minutes daily.

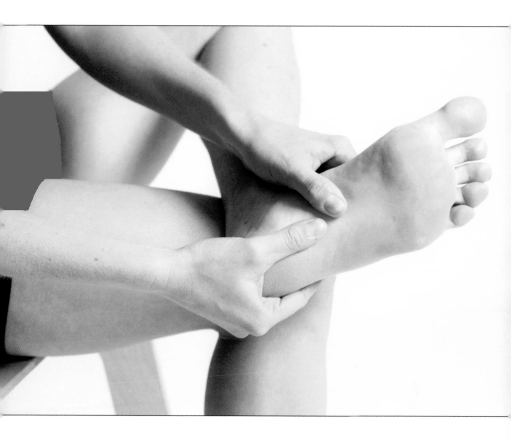

3. **Posterior tib** (muscle just on the inside of the ridge of the shin)—Apply pressure and flex and extend ankle to open tissue tightness. Do this 3–5 minutes daily.

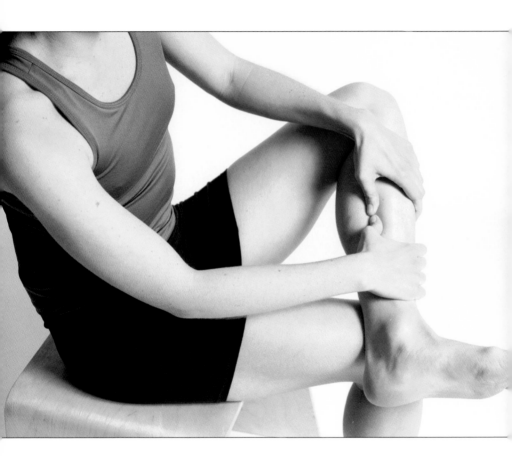

4. **Soleus** (the deep calf muscle)—Apply pressure and flex and extend ankle to open tissue tightness. Do this 3–5 minutes daily.

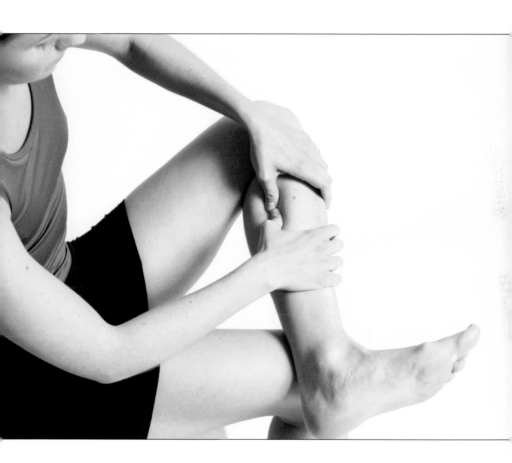

5. **Calf smash**—Place your calf on top of a foam roller or PVC pipe. Have a partner press firmly down on your calf as they rotate your leg in and out to break up small adhesions. This is pretty aggressive, but it's a great way to free up lingering tightness.

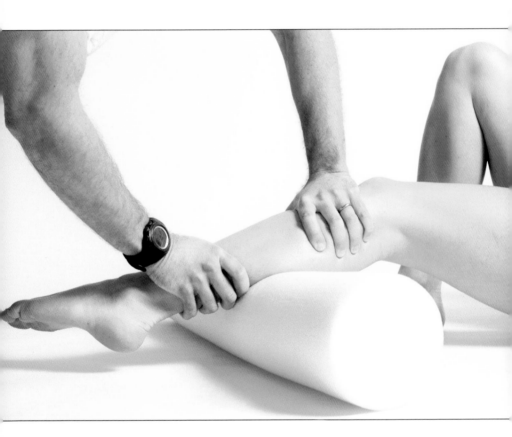

6. **Suprapatellar pouch**—
Place the LAX ball
just *above* the kneecap
and lie on your stom-
ach. Flex and extend
the knee. Highly effec-
tive for runners with
pain just below the
kneecap from infrapa-
tellar tendinosis and
fat pad impingement.

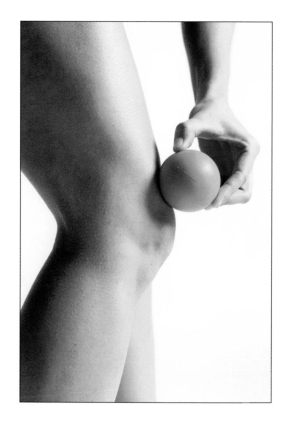

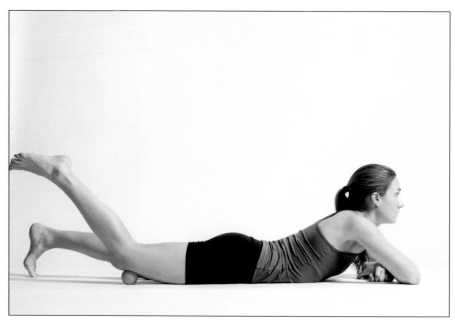

7. **Quad and IT band**—Almost everyone has rolled up and down on a foam roller, but it's even better to move the IT band across the adhered areas in the quad. Play around with the tilt of the body to find the most restricted areas, and flex and extend the knee to mobilize. If that isn't getting deep enough, use a LAX ball instead.

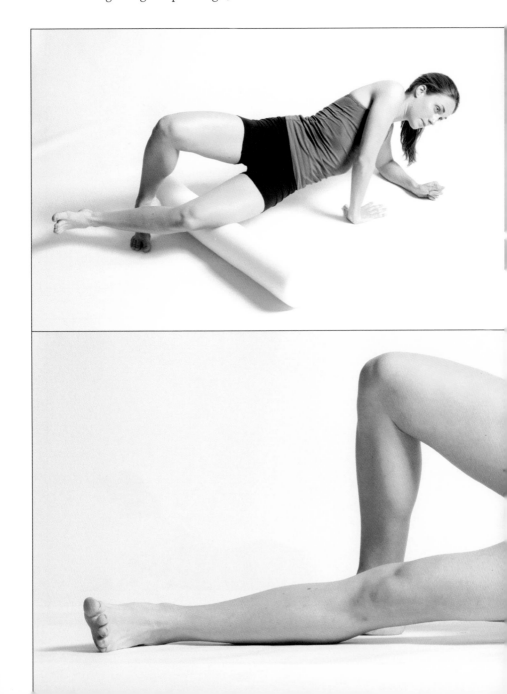

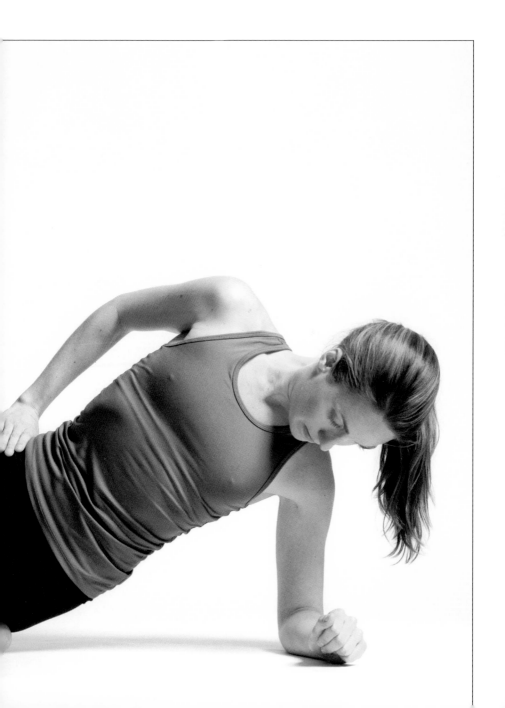

8. **Thoracic spine**—The mid back is stiff due to numerous rib attachments. Excessive curve here forces additional curve at the lumbar spine as well. Mobilizing this region is a great way to minimize strain on the low back and improve posture. Lie on your back so that the middle of your spine is weight-bearing on either a foam roller or a LAX ball. When you find overly stiff spots, work on them. You can also combine

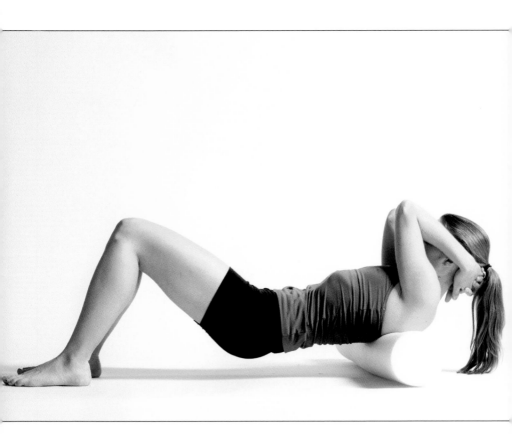

breathing to mobilize the ribs: inhale stiffens, exhale allows movement. Keep your head supported in your hands to minimize strain on
the neck and roll up and down to flatten out the thoracic spine. Do
this for a total of 3–5 minutes. Note—do not attempt this if you have
osteoporosis.

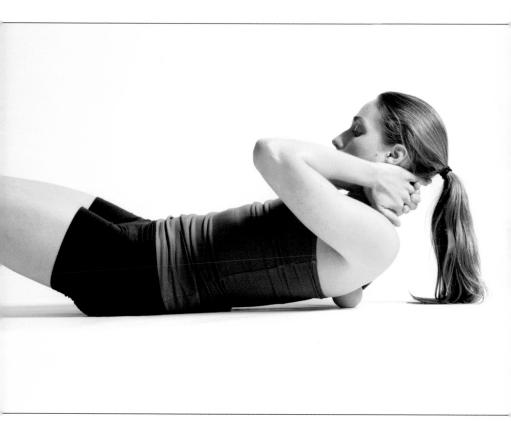

9. **Kneeling hip flexor**—We saved the best here for last. The stretch for the psoas is exactly the same as the test. Kneel down on one knee so that your thigh and shin remain vertical. Then tilt your pelvis backwards so that you spill your imaginary cereal bowl behind you. If you have trouble figuring this motion out, jump back inside the doorjamb to give you a better feel. If you want to kick it up a notch, you can rotate your hip slightly in (so rotate your foot slightly to the outside).

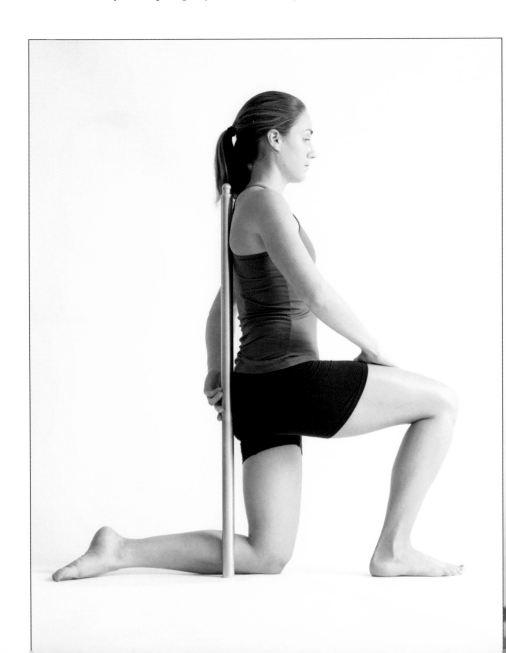

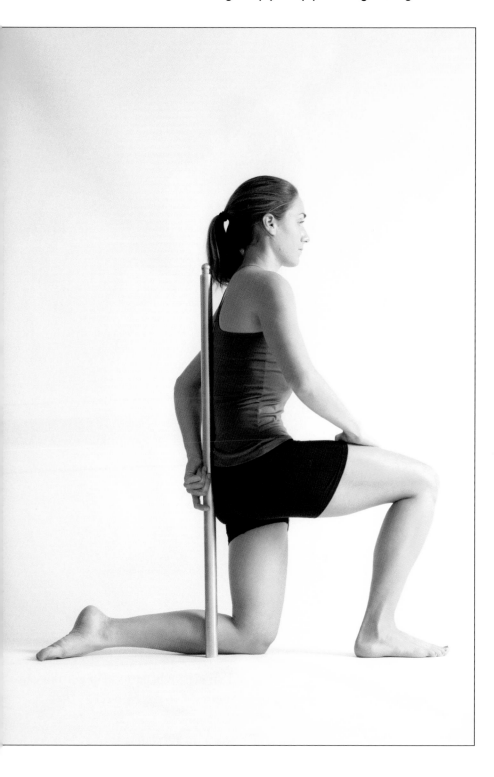

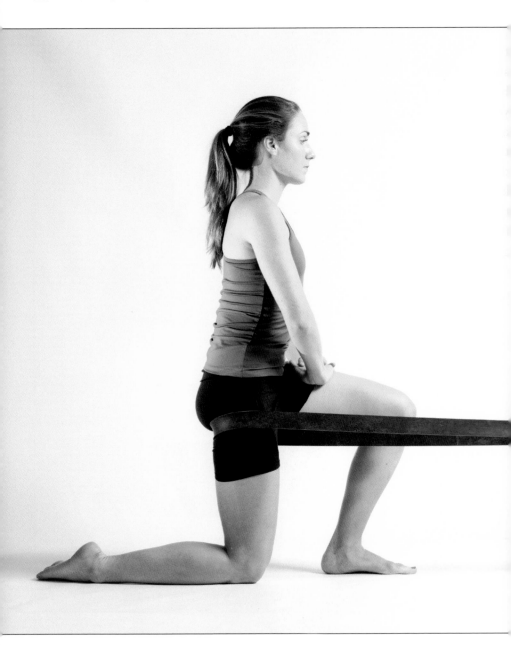

And for the most effective boost, add an elastic band to help get the capsule moving as well. Hold this for 3–5 minutes, 4–6 days a week.

If you want to try some soft tissue mobility work here as well, place your LAX ball right across the front of the hip joint. Lie down, bend your knee up and rotate the hip in and out for some deep tissue glide.

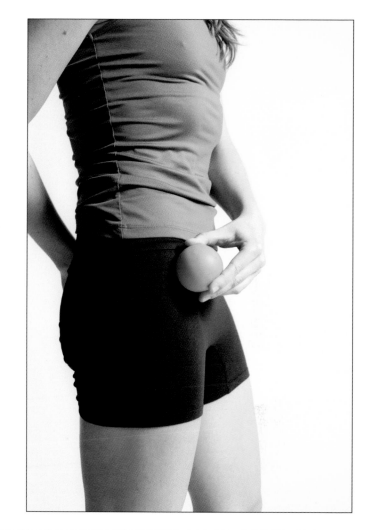

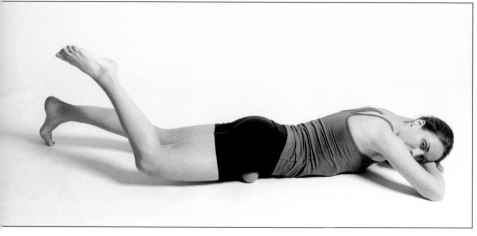

10. **Hamstring stretch**—Deficient hamstring mobility will force a flexed spine. A traditional hamstring stretch can be done by holding the leg up or by doing this stretch inside the doorway so that you can relax. Hold for 3–5 minutes.

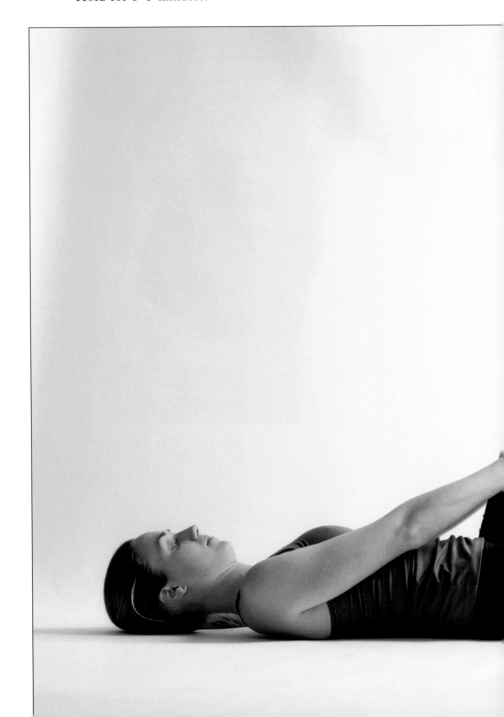

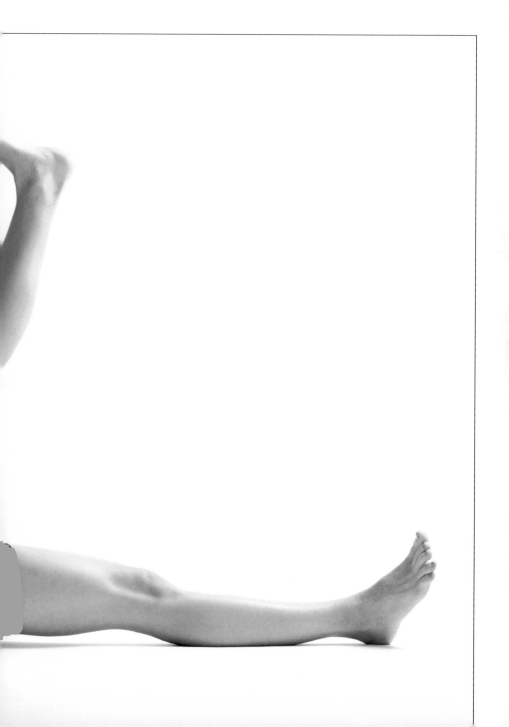

11. **Eccentric calf raise**—Raise up with both legs and down with one leg, 60 reps daily (typically done as 3 x 20 reps). Week 1: body weight to flat. Week 2: body weight to drop (done on stair or slant board). Week 3 through 6: progressively add weight in a backpack up to 45–55 pounds. These are done daily for the 6-week duration to repair chronic Achilles tendinopathy.

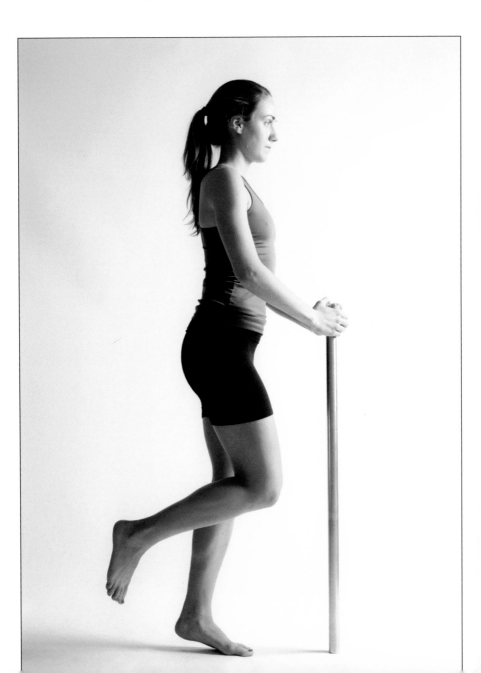

12. **Eccentric hamstrings** (band)—Eccentric contractions are the most beneficial thing you can do for chronic hamstring strains. Lie on your back with an elastic band tied to a support behind you. Insert your leg in the band and let it slowly pull your hip into flexion. When the hip is at your peak flexion, cross your free leg over the leg in the band and use it to help lower the banded leg to the ground. From an extended position, slowly let the band take you back to a flexed position. The amount of resistance should be moderate and allow you to complete 3 sets of 20 repetitions. These can be done daily for 6–8 weeks to remodel chronically strained hamstring tissues. Additionally, they can be done 2 times a week to help prevent future hamstring injury.

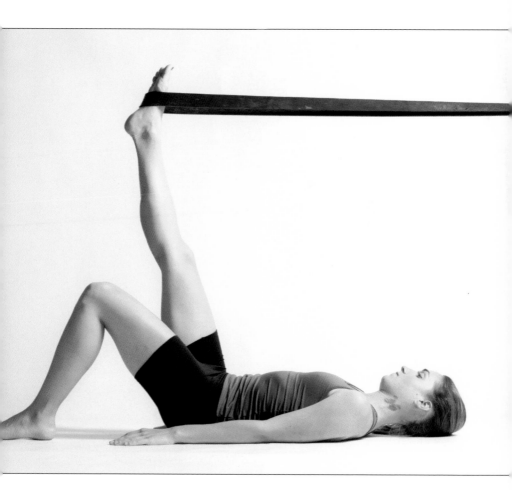

13. **Piriformis mobilization**—Stretching of the piriformis muscle is frequently recommended for sciatica. However, stretching can actually increase compression of the sensitive sciatic nerve over which it travels, making matters worse. So instead of stretching, it's more effective to mobilize this muscle. Place the LAX ball on the floor, and then lower yourself down on the ball so that it is on the back of the hip joint, and

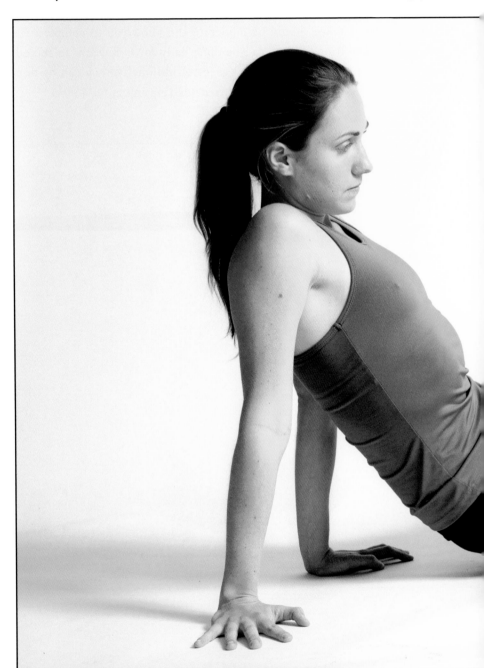

somewhat to the outside. Play with the amount of pelvic rotation until you feel maximum pressure on the piriformis. If you suffer from sciatic pain, seek out the exact spot where you feel the most discomfort—your symptoms will guide you to the best spot. Now adduct and abduct your hip slightly to free up the kinked tissue in the muscle belly.

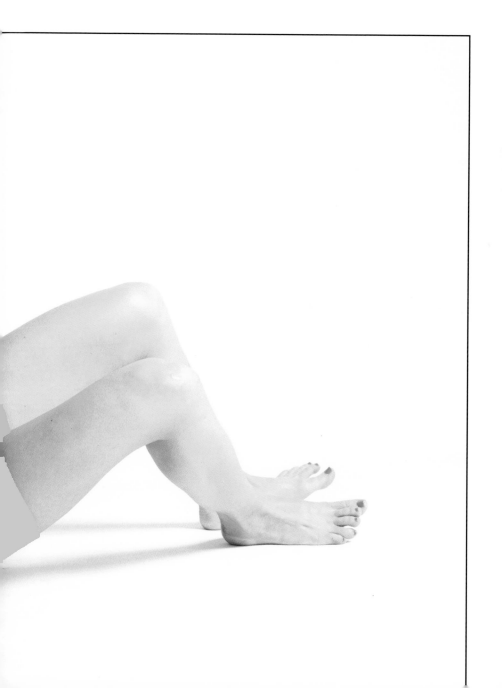

Get Smarter

The first step to improving your movements is to teach the right muscles to do their specific job.

1. **Core control**—Sit up straight or stand. Place your index finger on the bump in front of the pelvis near your belt, one on the left and one on the right. Then slide them straight up about 1 inch. This is the best location to feel the transversus without feeling too much of the obliques. Now make a face like you are about to say cheese for the camera. Your lips will pucker outward like you are blowing on a horn. We actually don't want to do this because you'll use the wrong muscles. So keep your teeth together, but let your lips relax. Next place your tongue up against the front of your teeth so it almost blocks the air from leaving your mouth. OK—now that you are set up take a regular inhalation and then a long slow exhalation. As you exhale, press your tongue against the front of your mouth. With the tongue providing pressure, the transversus has some pressure to push back against. If you are doing everything correctly, you should be able to feel the muscles poking outward into your fingers. While this breathing trick is a way to find your transverus, aim to tighten it at will. You should be able to uncouple your muscle control from your breathing.

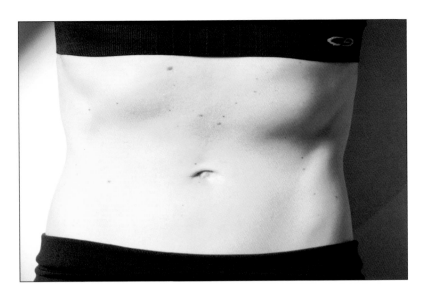

2. **Clamshells**—Improve your lateral hip stability from the muscles in the back of the hip, not the front. This exercise is frequently done wrong, making the benefits dissolve away. To ensure you get the most out of it, setup is critical. Begin by lying on your side with your torso and pelvis both perpendicular to the ground. Next, straighten the spine. When lying on our side, many of us slump into the floor. Slightly lift the belly up off the floor to create a stable core position. Now that you have established proper alignment, it's time to fire the glute medius. Squeeze your glutes tight like you have a quarter stuck between your butt cheeks. With your feet resting on each other, lift only the knee up until it's level with the hip. Lower the knee down keeping the glute contracted the entire time. Complete 100 reps daily.

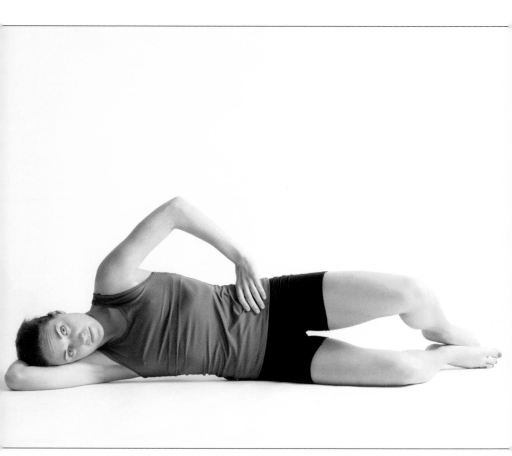

3. **Pigeon hip extension**—Isolate the glute max to extend the hip while keeping the spine stable. Get on the floor on your hands and knees. Tuck one leg underneath your chest (similar to the pigeon pose in yoga). Relax your upper body so you are resting your arms on your

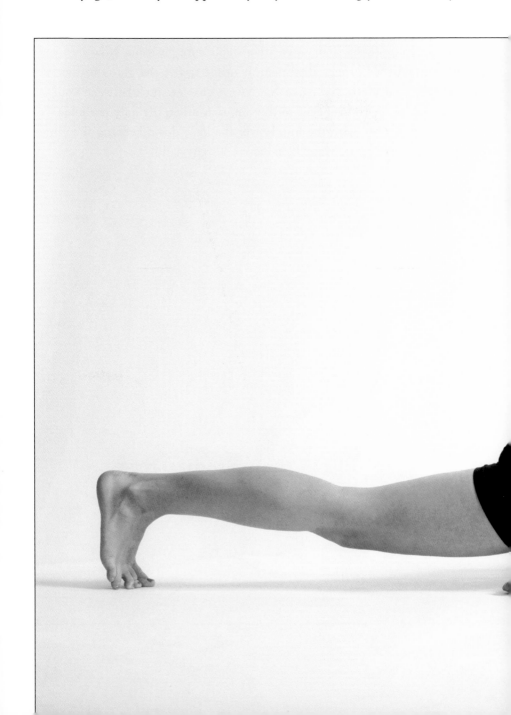

elbows. First, clench your butt cheeks together. While keeping your toes still on the ground, lift your knee straight off the floor. Hold for a count of one. Keeping glutes tight, return knee to the floor.

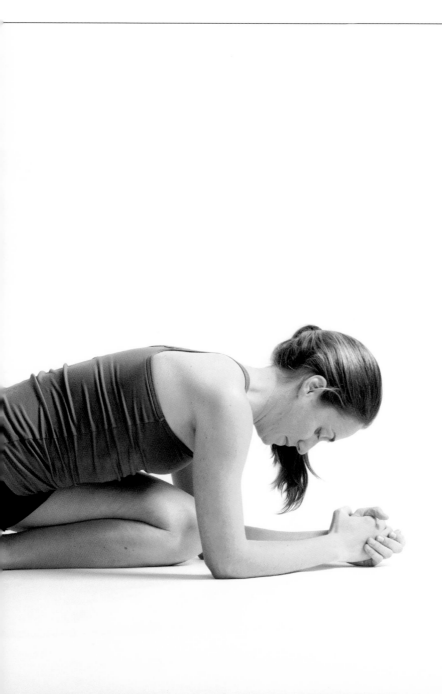

4. **Donkey kicks**—Learn the difference between hip extension and back extension. Begin on all fours with a 3–4 feet dowel across the back. Keeping the spine and dowel as still as possible, reach one leg back

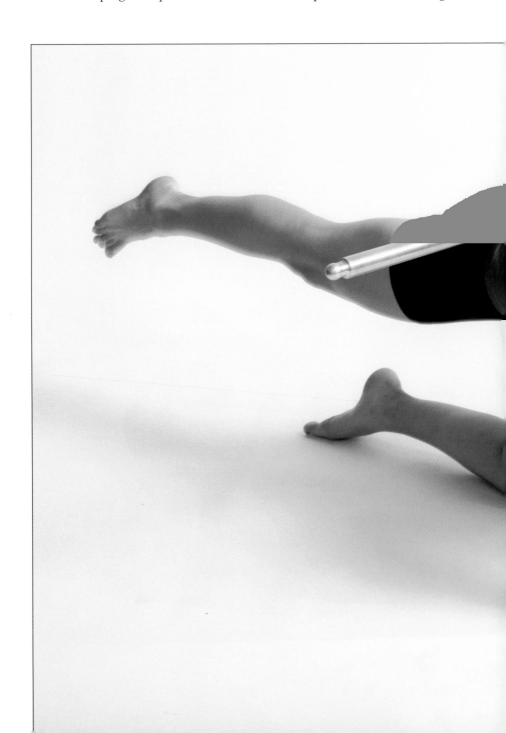

and slightly to the side. If you rock your body or the dowel excessively, make smaller movements until your control improves. Do 50 reps for each leg.

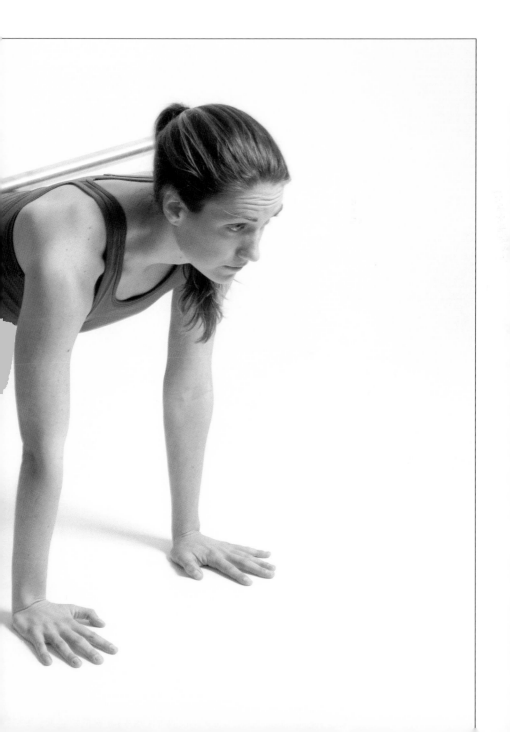

5. **Bridge/march bridge**—Initiate movement at the hip from the glutes, not the back. With your head, shoulders, and both feet on the floor, push up into a bridge position. While up, begin "marching"—alternate lifting each foot several inches off the ground, while keeping your pelvis steady and facing straight up. Do 3 sets of 20 marches (10 on each leg), with a short break between each set. If you have trouble "feeling"

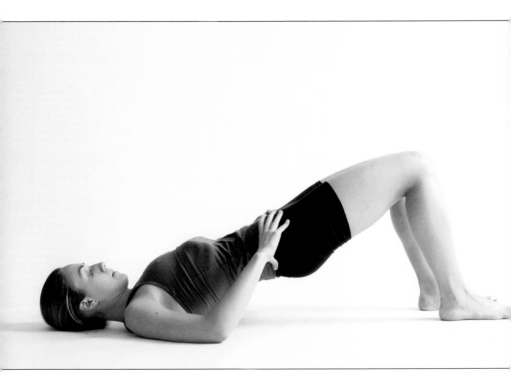

your glutes kick in or still find yourself tightening your low back, try this. Grab a partner and have them place their hands on the front of your pelvis and push very firmly down into the ground (almost all their body weight). When faced with this load, there is no way to cheat and bridge up with muscles in the low back.

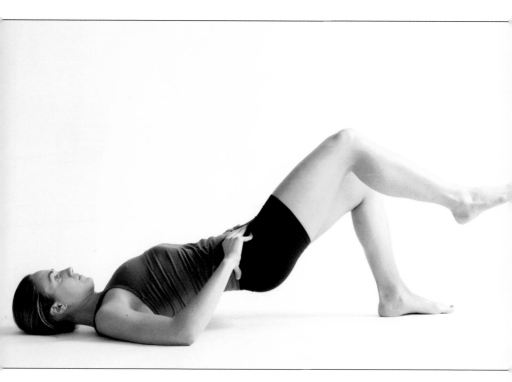

6. **Knee to chest bridge**—Improve glute max recruitment while eliminating the chance of arching the spine. Pull in your right knee, holding it against your chest. Keeping your head and shoulder blades on the floor, push up with your left leg into a bridge position while keeping your right leg against you. Push up, keeping the pelvis level, then lower yourself down. Do 12 to 15, then switch legs. Do three sets on each side.

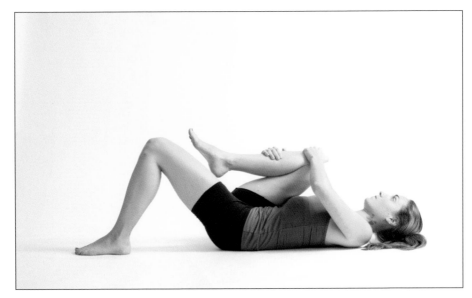

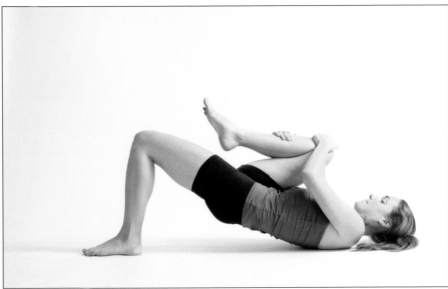

7. **Big toe isolation**—The toe should provide the majority of the stability in the foot. Let's get yours working. Sit down with your foot flat on the floor and equal pressure across the ball of the foot. Reach down and lift the end of your big toe off the floor. From here, push the toe straight down, keeping the middle joint straight, as you slowly resist this motion with your hand. This will teach you to isolate the big toe from the little toes. If you find that you want to bend the joint in the toe, you can place a finger on top to block it until you learn to move correctly. When you can do this, the test becomes the exercise. Practice for 3–5 minutes daily for 1–2 weeks.

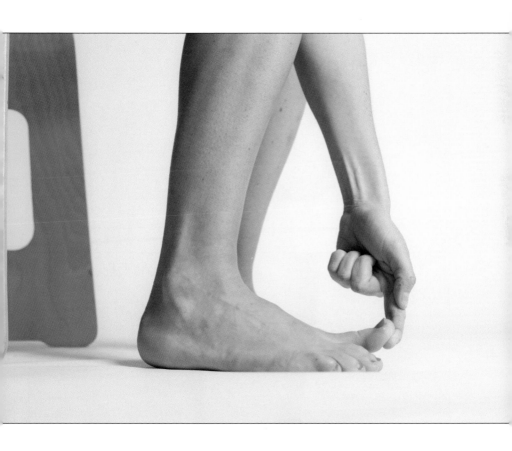

8. **Toe yoga**—For foot coordination. Simply try to raise/lower the little toes and big toe independently of each other to improve coordination. Do this several times a day until easily mastered. Since it's targeting a change in control and not strength, improvements are rapid—usually noticeable in a few days to two weeks. Do this daily for 3–4 minutes per foot until it is easy.

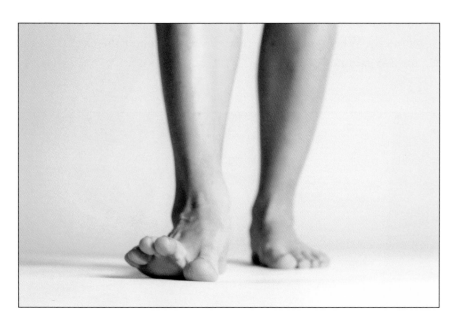

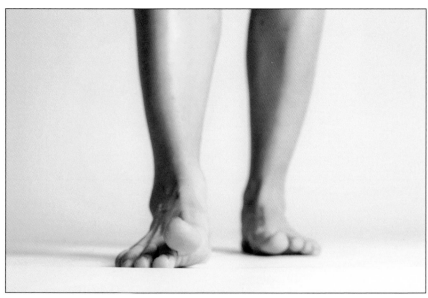

9. **Single-leg balance**—Develop a solid contact point in your foot. To use the forefoot for balance, you first need to have weight equally over your forefoot and rearfoot. Too many runners have a habit of standing in the backseat with weight over the heel. To find the correct position, place one hand on your belly button and one hand on your sternum. Drop forward slightly at the waist (not the ankle and knee) until you feel weight equally distributed over the forefoot and rearfoot. With your big toe firmly pressed into the ground (you did pass the toe yoga test, right?), try to stand quietly for 30 seconds at a time. Imagine a triangle between the inside ball of the foot (first metatarsal), the end of the

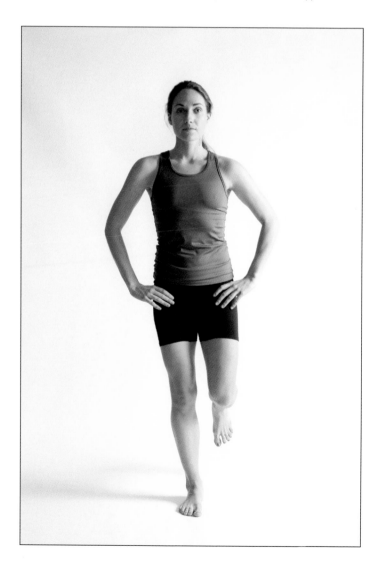

big toe, and the outside ball of the foot (fifth metatarsal) that remains in solid contact with the floor. Do this with eyes open and closed; try rotating back and forth or throwing a ball with someone or against a wall to increase the difficulty. Balance training is best done in short spurts of 20–30 seconds, multiple times a day rather than in one 10–minute block. You can do this when brushing your teeth, making lunch, or pouring your cereal. Most runners are surprised at both how bad their balance is and how quickly it can improve. This can go from poor to excellent in a few weeks since it involves training the neuromuscular system.

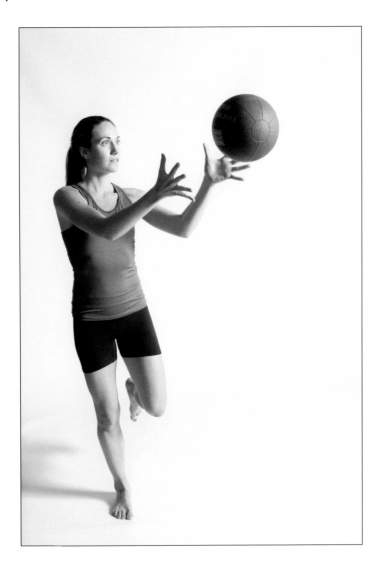

10. **Standing hip extension**—Activate your hip extensors while keeping the spine stable. Stand up so that the front of your thighs are up against a table. Place one hand on the back and one hand on the small of the back. Bend one knee so it is 90 degrees. Push the foot into an imaginary wall behind you without any increase in arch or tightness in the lower back . . . hip extensors. Do 30 reps to learn proper movement.

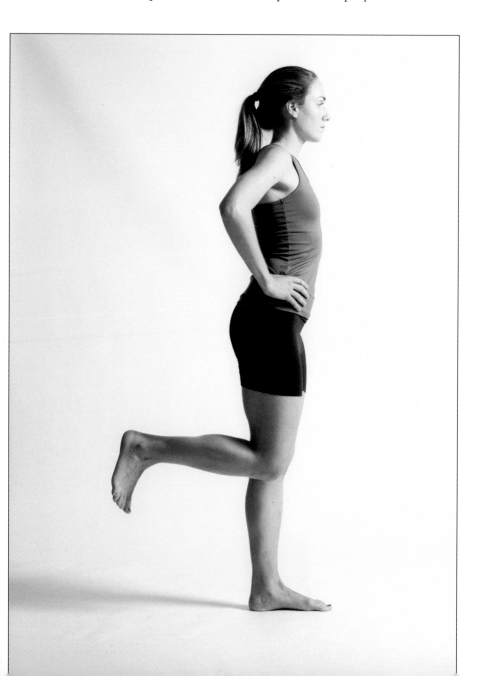

11. **Chair of death**—OK, this exercise won't really kill you, but it will completely rewire the way you move. Take the emphasis off of your quads and shift it to your glutes. Grab a stick (pipe, broom, yardstick) so that it is touching your tailbone, your back, and the middle of your head. Stand facing a chair. The front of your knees should actually be touching the chair. As you squat down, move your butt backwards, just like you are doing the "hover" over a toilet. The most important thing

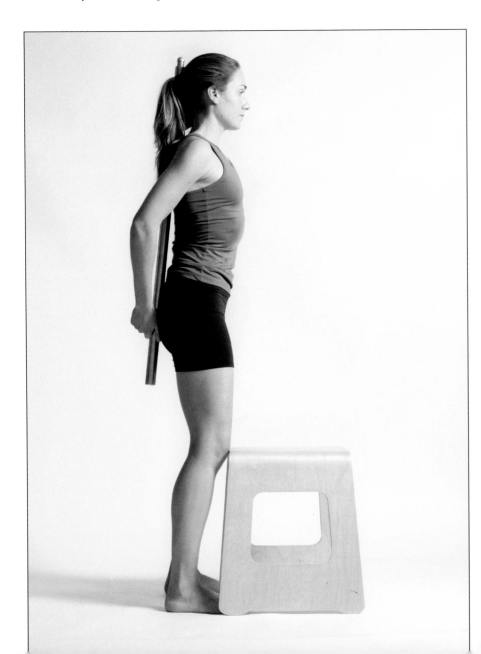

is to make sure that the bar doesn't come off the back of your body and that you hinge from your hip. It's OK to lean the trunk forward here when starting. Your first goal is to be able to squat to parallel (horizontal thighs) and the long-term goal is to be able to lower well beyond parallel (almost to the ground). As your glute strength improves, you'll be able to keep your torso more upright and lower down further. Do 3 sets of 10 reps.

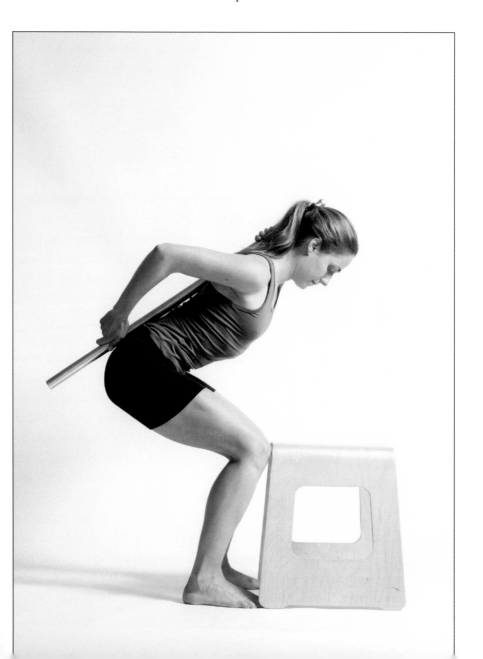

Should I do my foot balance exercises in my bare feet or shoes? Proprioception is the fastest information that gets relayed to your brain. The nerves that conduct this information are large and very well insulated to ensure that information you "sense" from the body reaches your brain faster that you can see or hear it. So if the goal is to "tune" this position sense, it makes "sense" that the foot should be on flat firm ground so that you can learn to pick up on subtle differences in foot position. This sense should take priority over all else. Wearing shoes places us on a mushy unstable surface that makes it harder to sense joint position. Firm surfaces help wake up the feet—get those shoes off to maximize your time invested.

Get Stronger

So you've done a few weeks of retraining. Movements that seemed quite foreign now feel more natural. If they don't, you should stick around the Phase 1 exercises a bit longer. When you know you're moving correctly, it's time to bump your efforts up a notch. Some of these exercises are hard! Never compromise your form quality to hit a specific quantity. The sets and reps suggested are goals and not necessarily where you should begin on day one.

12. **Rocker board**—The single best way to improve your foot strength is to use a rocker board. First, tilt the board so that it is at 45 degrees to your body. The reason for this is that the axis of pronation in the foot is closer to this orientation than when it is straight across. You want to make your training functional. Since the only way you can control the board is by using your foot, it's critical to keep the "triangle" of the inside and outside ball of the foot and the end of your big toe firmly down on the board. While standing with good posture, touch the toe side of the board down to the ground, then the heel side. This is one rep. Repeat for 2 set of 20 reps. Then rotate the board 90 degrees so that you are working the opposite 45-degree axis (on the same foot) so that you complete 2 sets of 20 reps in *each* 45-degree axis on each foot several days a week. If you need support, feel free to stick one finger on a wall. It's better to get help and control what you can than to flop about aimlessly.

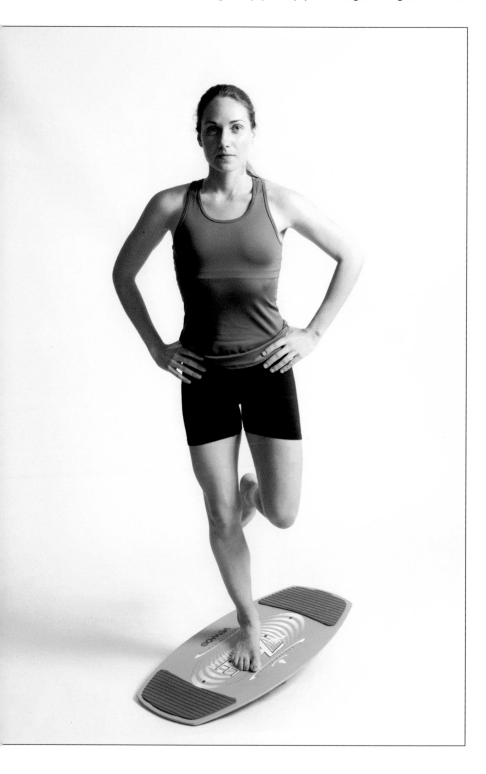

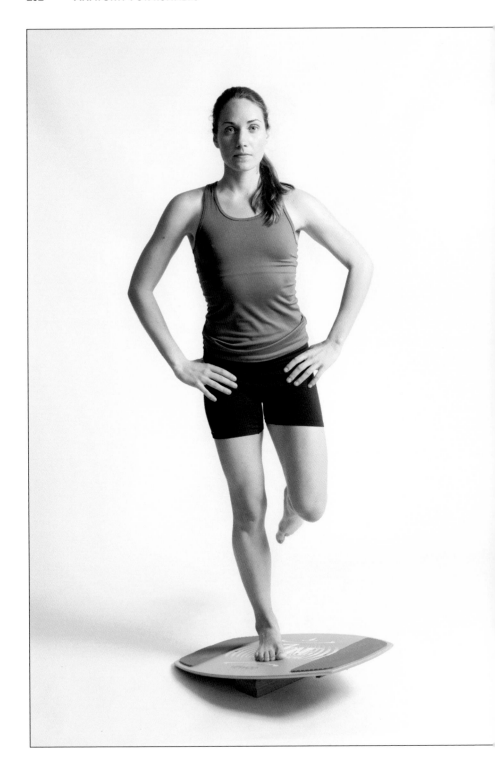

13. **Rocker squats**—Help bring the body back to midline. This exercise encourages multiple plane stability at the core, hips, and feet. Stand on rocker board with feet slightly wider than shoulder width. With hands on hips, squat down keeping knees over the second toes. Use a mirror to make sure that knees don't crash to the inside. Do 3 sets of 10 reps.

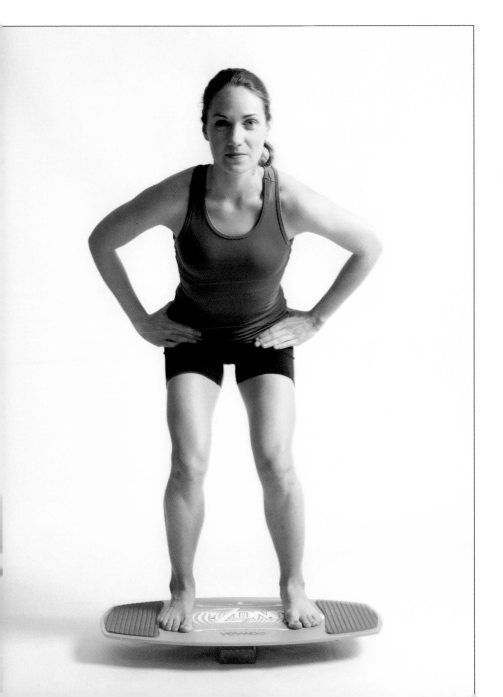

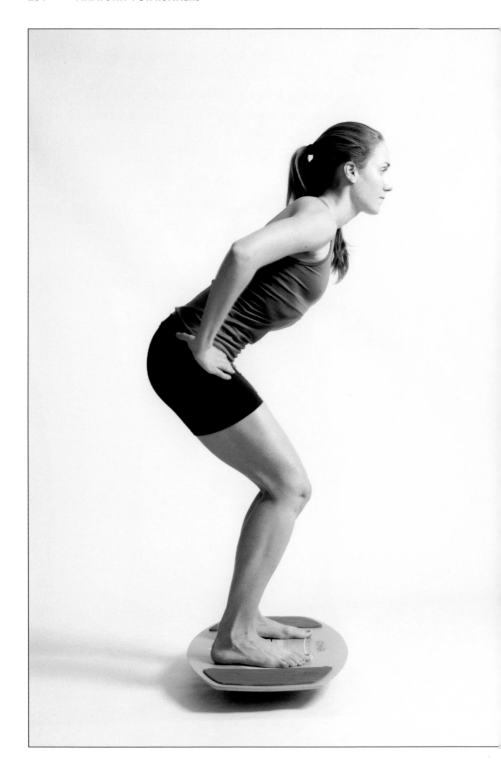

14. **Hip hike**—Improve your lateral hip stabilization. Stand on one leg with your hands on hips. Without shifting your trunk, drop the opposite side of the pelvis down, return it back to level, and then raise it up. You should feel this working in the hip on the leg you are standing on. If you feel this more in front of the hip, it means your posture is likely slumped in the backseat. Drop the chest forward slightly and repeat and you should feel this more in the outside of the butt cheek. Do 3 sets of 10 reps.

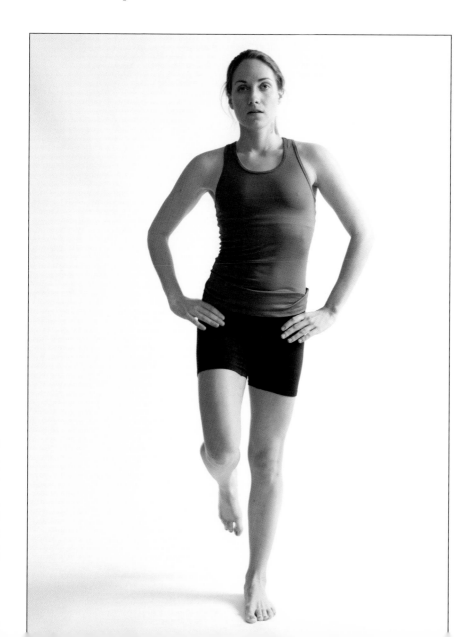

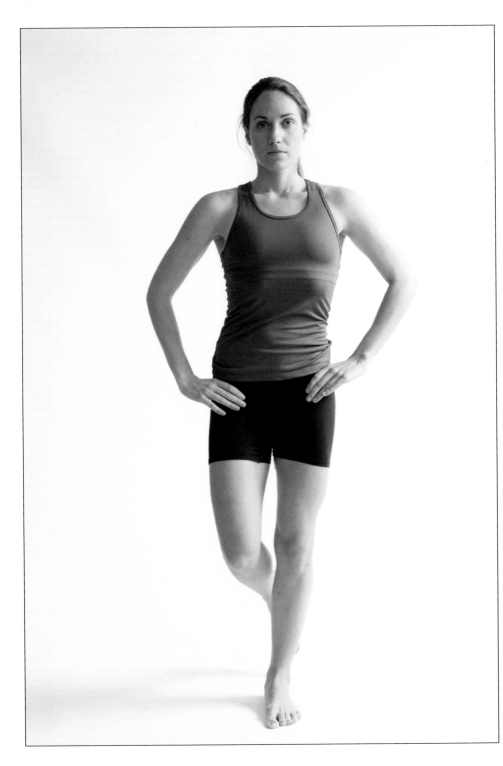

15. **T-ball triad**—This exercise has three parts to improve hip extension in a very running-specific range of motion. Phase 1: Lie on your back with your legs up on the ball. While keeping your core muscles tight, squeeze an imaginary quarter between your butt cheeks and raise your hips up off the floor. Lower down while keeping the butt tight throughout the range. You need to control your motion, not just flop up and down using momentum. Repeat for a set of 10.

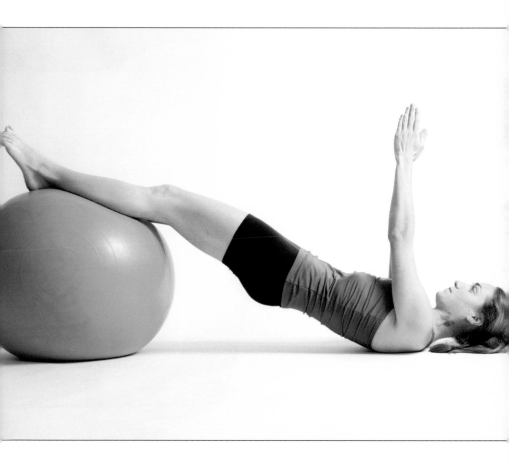

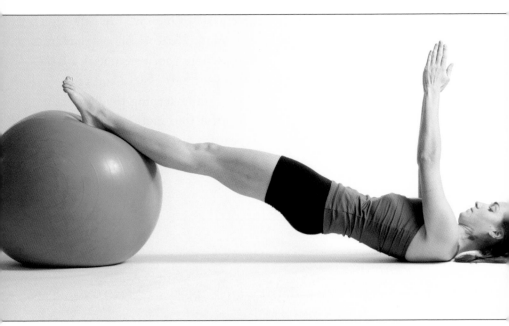

Phase 2: This time extend your legs straight out with the ball underneath your feet. While keeping the butt tight, bridge up and down for a set of 10.

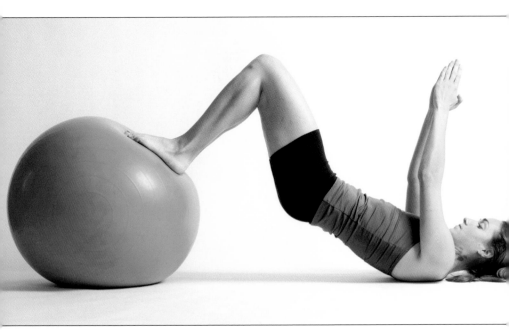

Phase 3: Just like Phase 2, except when you are up, curl the ball towards your butt while keeping hips high and do 3 sets of 10 reps.

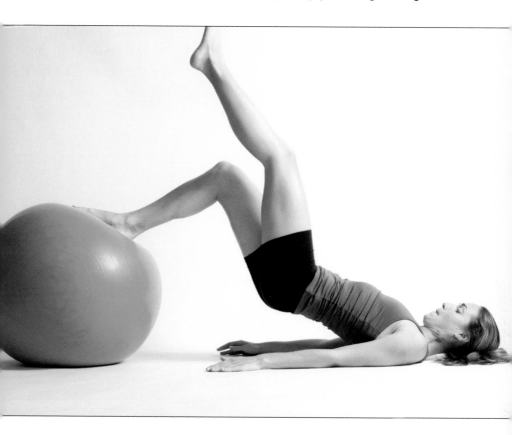

You can adjust difficulty with your arm contact. Arms flat on the ground provide more stability than arms pointing up at the sky. And when you are really ready for a challenge, go through this entire sequence on one leg.

16. **Swiss ball walk-out**—Improve core control and shoulder stability for posture. Arrange yourself in a plank position with the Swiss ball underneath your feet. Walk continually back and forth for 30 seconds. Do 3 reps. Make sure to keep the spine straight without excessive arch or excessive pike up to the sky.

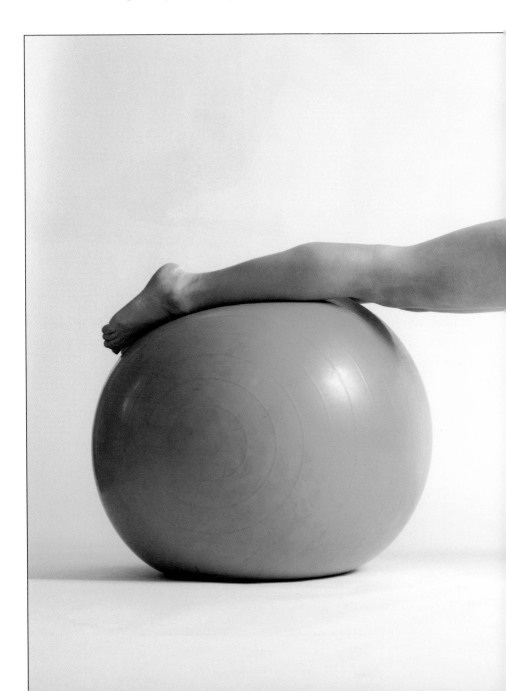

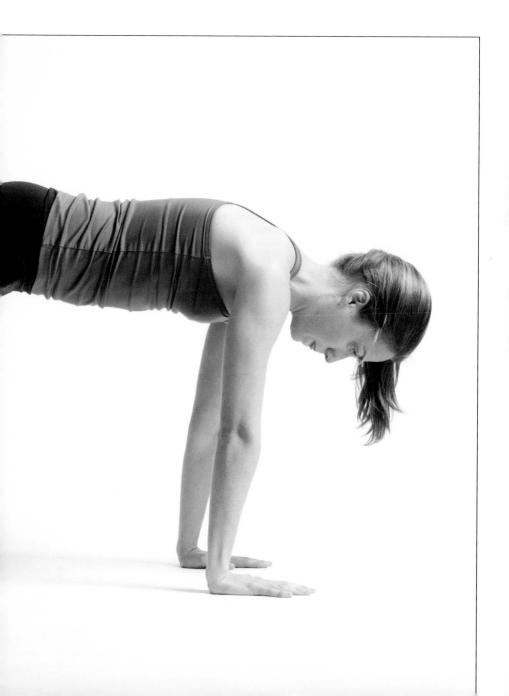

17. **Swiss ball lateral walk**—Improve core control and shoulder stability for posture. Arrange yourself in a plank position with the Swiss ball underneath your feet. Pretend you are balancing a full glass of water between your shoulder blades. Walk your hands slowly sideways and then back to the other side for 30 seconds. Do 3 sets of 10 reps.

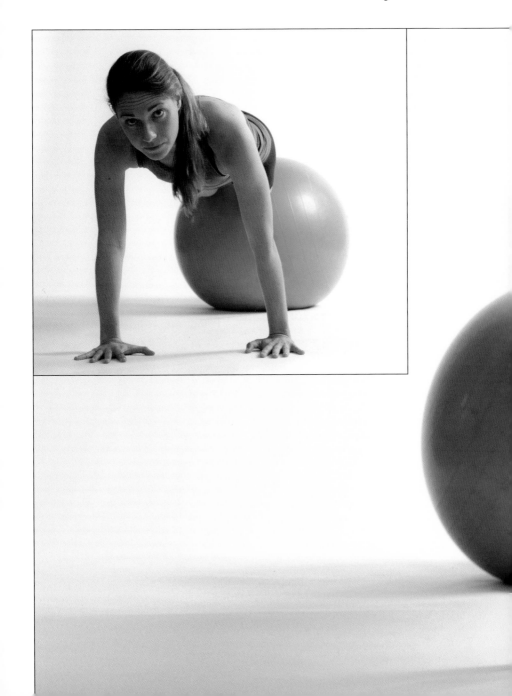

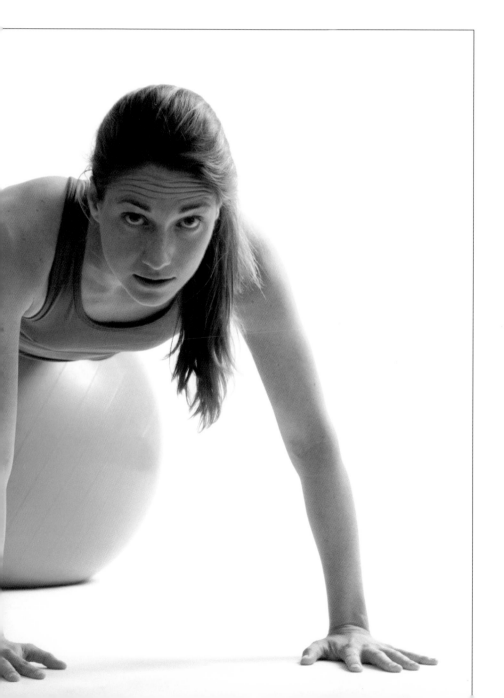

18. **Swiss ball pike**—Challenge your core stabilization while improving your shoulder strength for good posture. Position yourself in a plank position with feet on the ball. Pike your hips upward just like a diver. Make sure to keep the spine straight. The majority of the motion should be from your hips, not your back. Do 3 sets of 10 reps.

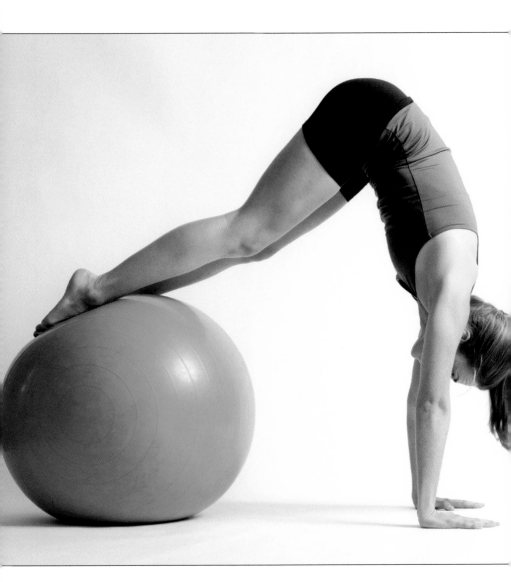

19. **Swiss ball rock 'n' roll**—Hands and knees is a great position to improve core activation, and the wobble of the ball kicks it up a level. Standing behind the ball, bend over so your hands and knees are on the ball. Gently roll forward so you are basically kneeling on a Swiss ball. Show the ball who is boss! Next, slowly rock the ball forward/backward or side to side while you maintain control. As your stability improves on your hands and knees, walk the ball down the room, out the door, and up the hill. This is a great competitive stabilization exercise for running teams.

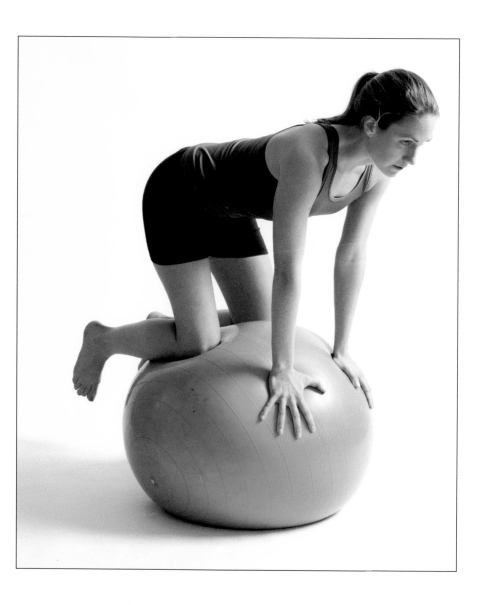

20. **Swiss ball hip extension**—While keeping a stable position on the ball, extend one leg out behind you. Tough? Sure. Important? Yes. This is the type of move that helps you maintain postural control during full race efforts. Do 3 sets of 8 reps for each leg.

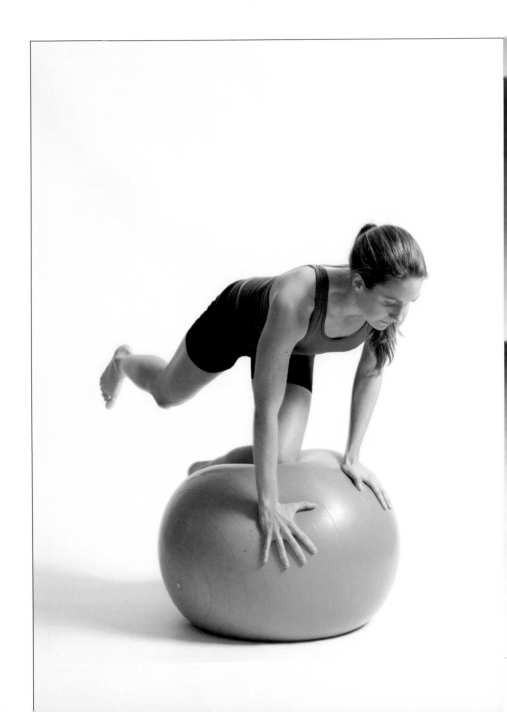

21. **Single-leg dead lift**—The best way to strengthen your glute max. Begin on both legs with a dowel along the back. Bend forward making sure that you keep the dowel firmly on the body. This will force you to move from the hip and not the spine. As you return to standing, emphasize pushing the pelvis forward to help activate the glute. Repeat this a few times to get the motion down. When you are ready, we'll move to the real exercise which does this same motion on one leg. Keep the pelvis level and stable when flexing forward. Keeping the opposite leg extended behind you will help counterbalance the body. To come up, simply push the pelvis forward to come up from the glutes. Ensure you keep equal pressure across the ball of the foot when doing these to improve your stance control. Do 3 sets of 10 reps.

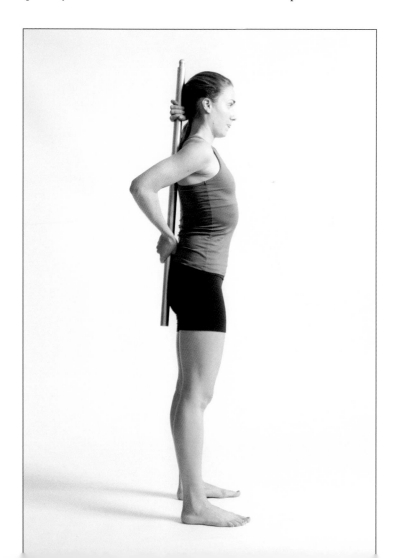

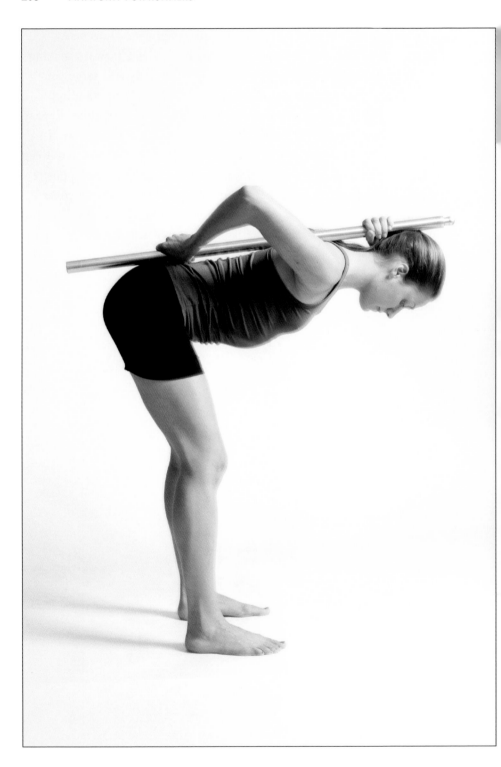

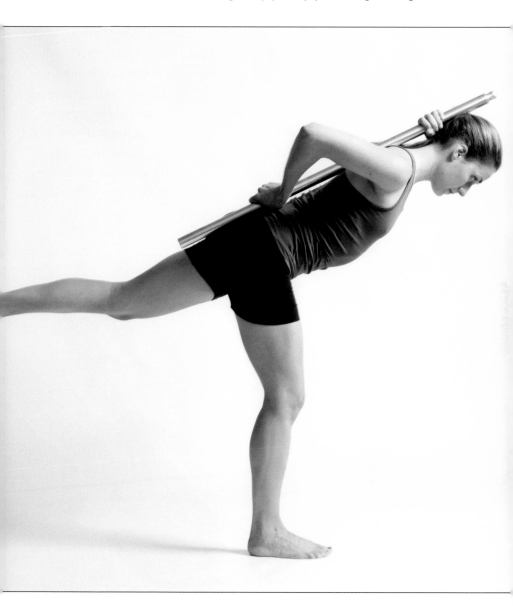

22. **Twisting lunge**—Improves rotational stabilization of the hips while encouraging a glute dominant movement pattern. Stand with a dowel across shoulders. One leg is resting on chair/bench well behind you (needs to be further back than you may think), and the opposite leg is slightly in front of the body. Now lunge down and backwards like you are sitting on a chair behind you so that 60–70 percent of your body weight transfers to the back leg. The lead shin should remain completely vertical and not move forward at all. Once down in the lunge, rotate shoulders right 45 degrees, then to left 45 degrees, then center, and back up. This is one rep. Do 3 sets of 10 reps for each leg.

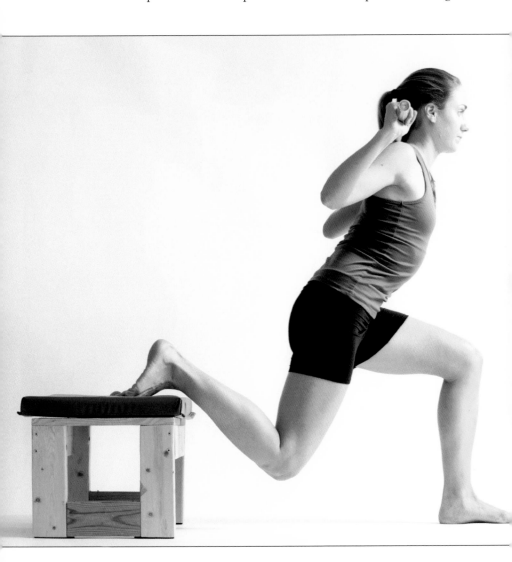

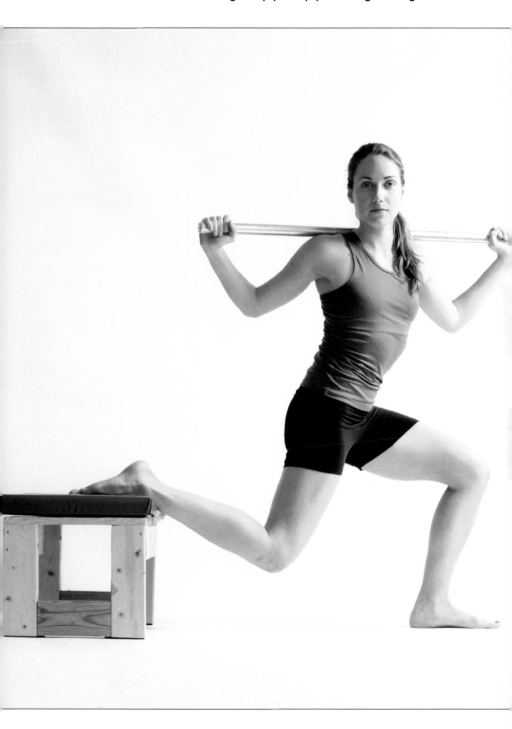

23. **Swiss ball Russian twist**—Very high level multiplane core and hip stability. Place your hands on a bench and the ball under your feet in a plank position. Lift one foot off the ball. Rotate it under and across

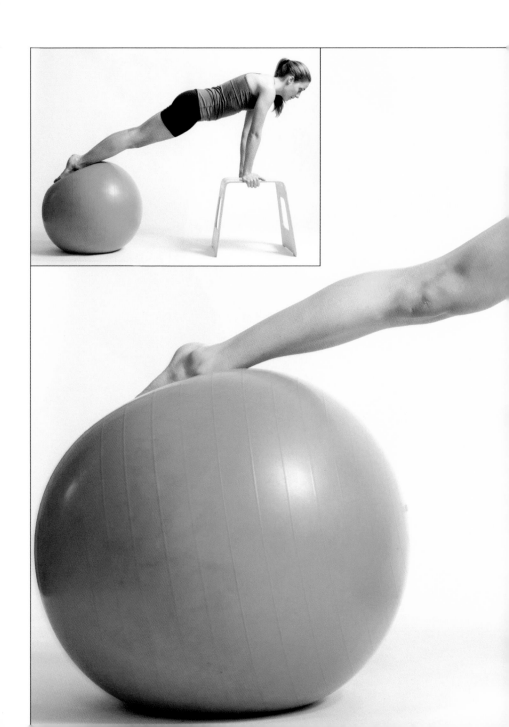

your body and back—look out for any tightness or arch in the lower back. Complete 3 sets of 8 twists for each leg.

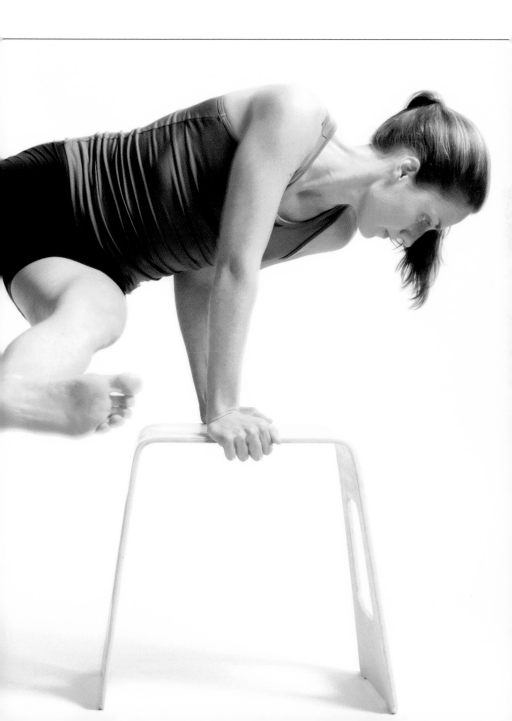

24. **T-Ball torso rotations**—This is an advanced posture exercise. Some amount of rotation between the upper body and lower body is normal when running. However, excessive arch in the low back is not. Kneel on the T-ball with your thighs straight up and down to take excess pressure off the quads. Then reach your arms out to the side at 90 degrees to the body. While keeping your pelvis and eyes forward, rotate your arms and torso 90 degrees. If you rotate around your spine, your weight will stay over the ball. However, if you arch as you twist, your body weight will shift and you'll be kicked off the ball. Do 3 sets of 20 reps for each side.

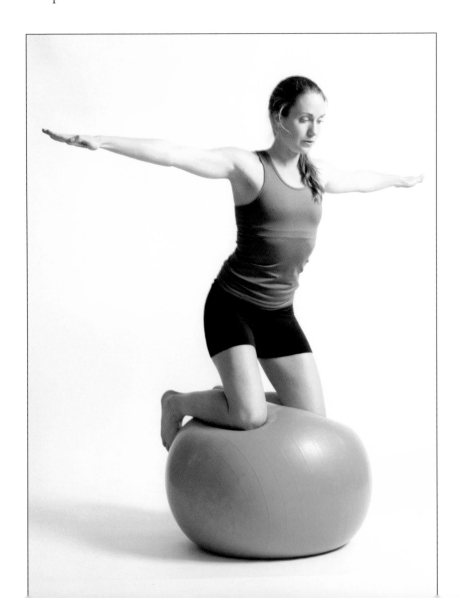

25. **Rotisserie chicken**—For rotational hip and core control. Place your ball in the corner for additional stability. Lie with one leg on the ball and one slightly off the ball. Place your hands on your hips and bridge up so the body is straight. As if you are a chicken on a spit, rotate the opposite side up, back to center, and down. The key here is rotating from the hip, making sure to have absolutely no arch or tightness in the back. If any tightness is felt in the low back, drop the pelvis lower and try to rotate again. Do 3 sets of 10 reps.

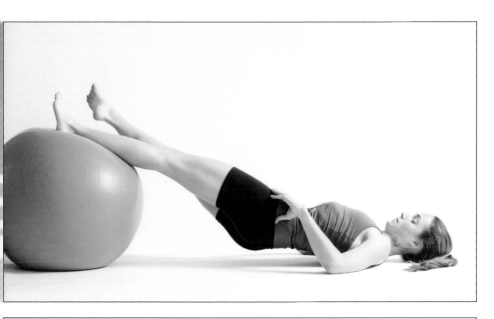

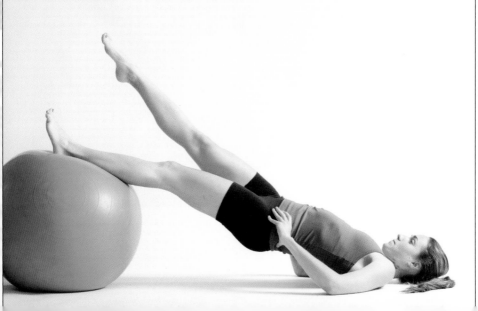

26. **Side-lying hip bridge**—Strengthens the hip abductors while training proximal core control. While lying on your side and top leg up on Swiss ball (or chair/bench), push the foot down into the ball so that the entire body rises off the floor while keeping the spine stable. Do 3 sets of 10 reps.

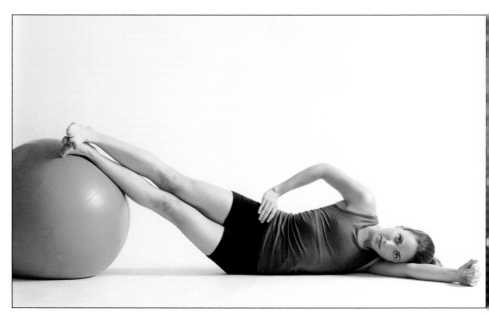

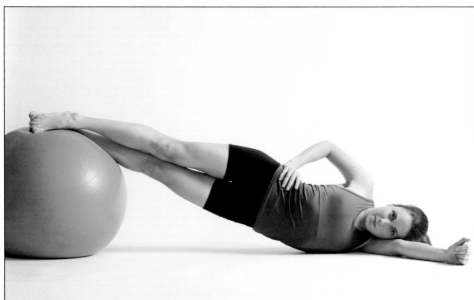

27. **Side-lying hip adduction**—Strengthens hip adductors while requiring proximal core control. While lying on your side and top leg up on Swiss ball (or chair/bench), pull the foot in towards midline so that the entire side of the body raises up off of the floor. Make sure the spine stays straight and stable. Do 3 sets of 10 reps.

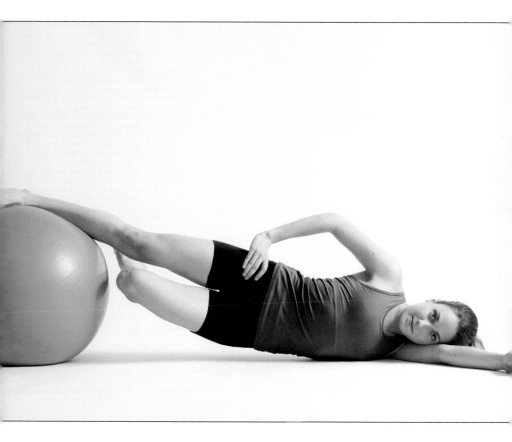

Improving the Spring

The key is maintaining proper form with explosive power. Know when you are ready to transition these into your routine. These are best done on days when you are not fatigued. Ideally, this would be at two days or more away from your speedwork sessions.

28. **Ninja squat jumps**—This will improve two key aspects: 1) Teach you to absorb the stresses of landing to minimize high loading rates that can cause compressive stress fractures, and 2) Develop explosive force during stance. When starting, only jump up and then step down since the goal is landing as softly as possible. You should literally not hear a sound when you land. Overly hard landings indicate poor shock absorption strategy. After you've learned to land softly, jump both up and down. Stand right against the box you are jumping up on. Begin with a box about midshin high, and progress until you can do a box midthigh height. Aim for 10–30 jumps, 1–2 days a week.

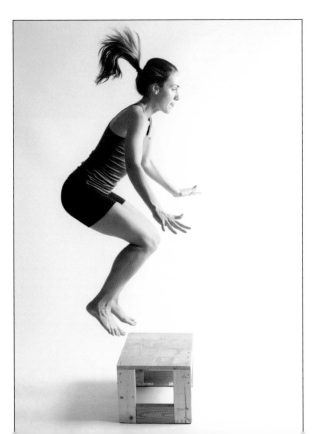

29. **Lateral jumps**—Jumping sideways is a great way to recruit your lateral hip stabilizers at a much higher intensity. These can be tough—but the pay off is big. Stand alongside any type of object from one inch to mid-shin height. Jump over sideways for 10 reps, staying on the ground as little time as possible. Aim for 3–4 sets. Think quick feet.

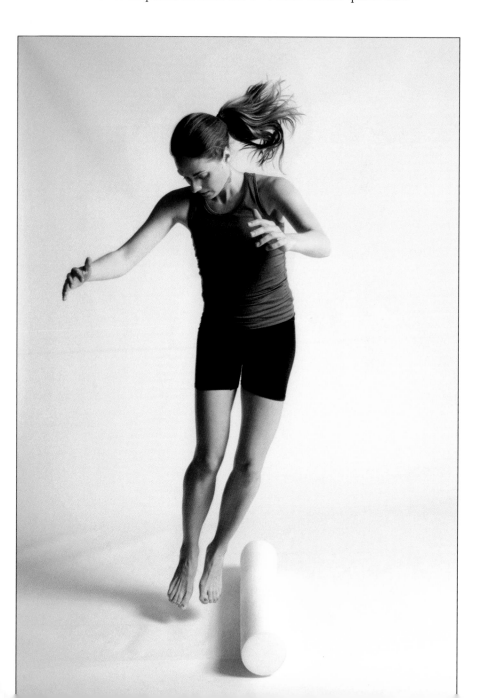

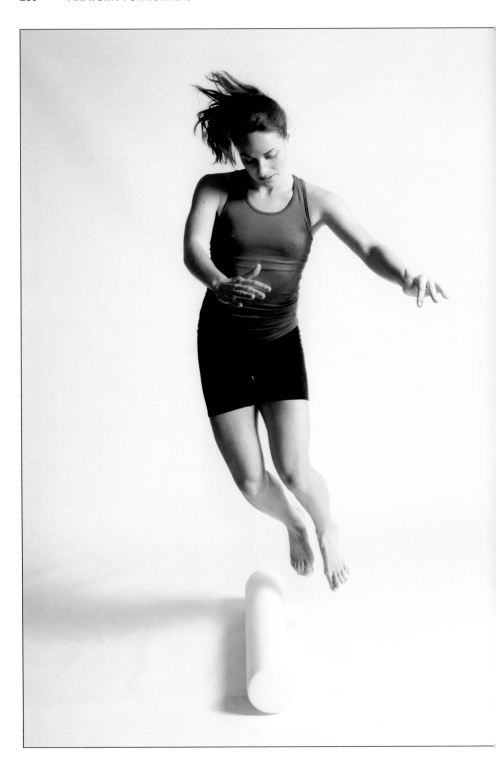

30. **4-Square**—Basically a single-leg hop with quick direction changes added in. While it's nice to have a square grid drawn out on the floor in tape, its not 100 percent necessary. You can do these on a tile floor to simulate the grid, or simply eyeball landmarks on the ground for spatial awareness. Jump up to each corner of the box as quickly as possible for 10 seconds straight and do 2–6 reps.

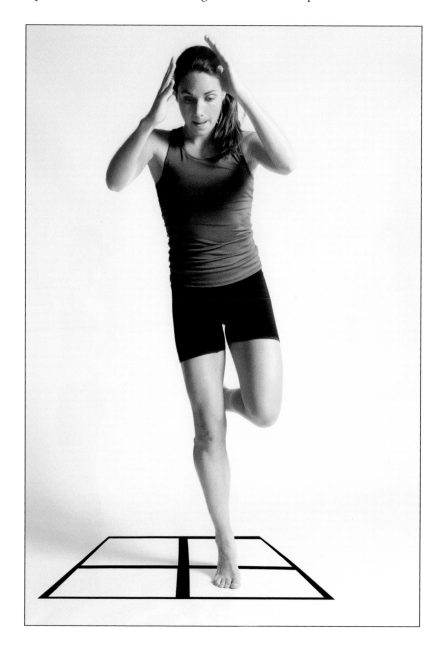

31. **Heel lift drill**—Avoid the tendency to lift and reach the foot out in front of you when running, as shown below. Instead, place your hands on your hips to help maintain your neutral posture alignment. Look back to the vertical compression test for reference. While keeping the spine in neutral, lift the heel up off the ground without flexing your hip forward. You'll notice that the muscles doing the work are your

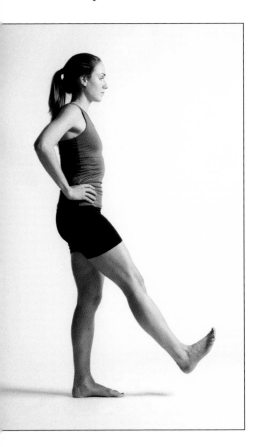

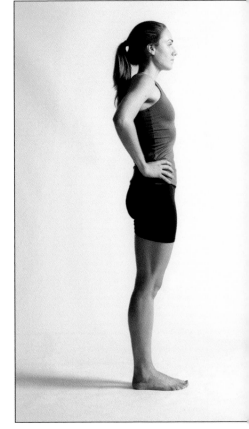

glutes and hamstrings, not your hip flexors. Alternate between the left and right legs, getting faster and faster until you are practically running in place. Then move backwards and forwards several steps at a time to cue you to land with your foot close to the body. Try this drill for a few minutes, both prior to and during your runs, to change your habits. The goal is to run from the butt, not from the hip flexors and calves.

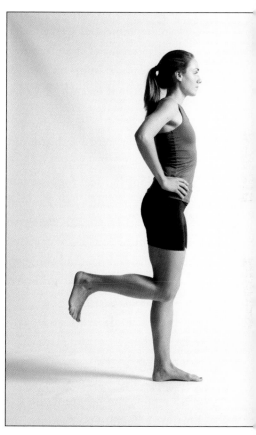

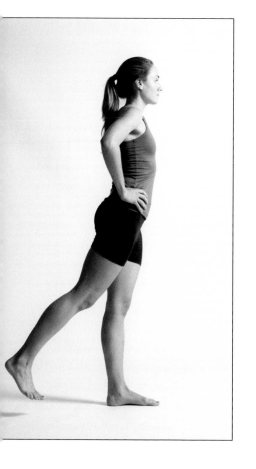

32. **Olympic lifts**—Squats, dead lifts, power cleans, clean and jerks, push-press. Again, get someone knowledgeable on technique to show you the ropes.

33. **Metronome jump rope**—Jumping rope, with a little help from technology, can dramatically improve your explosiveness. Since jumping rope is basically a plyometric with some movement skill training, this may be one of the most powerful ways to improve your contact time. Grab your smartphone and download the metronome program of you choice (typically free). Set it somewhere between 175-220 beats per minute, and try to keep up! Jump on two feet and also on one foot while cranking that rope. You'll learn how to be explosive and refine your coordination.

When you were a kid, you did lots of different stuff. Each time you moved around, you learned to refine your movement skills, improve your coordination, and feel for a certain activity. And sometimes you screwed up and tripped, or didn't kick the ball through the uprights on the football field or whatever. The point is that you tried, and kept trying, and kept refining your control of your body. Somewhere along the line, you made the decision to focus on running. And somewhere along that line, you stopped doing other stuff. And you lost skills. You became less of an athlete.

Whose fault is this? Part of it is yours, part of it is your grade school and high school's fault, and part of it is your coach's. Whoa! Did I ruffle some feathers? Let's explain. Many years ago, I treated a seven-year-old baseball player. He came to see me for back pain he's had for almost six months. Yes—a seven-year-old with chronic low back pain! It took me all of 45 seconds to pinpoint the source of his pain over the last six months. This kid's posture was awful. I mean really, really bad. He stood by placing all of the load on his joint structure and for all intents and purposes disconnected his neuromuscular system from controlling anything. He was completely clueless as to how to change his posture. There is a lot of load going through the spine at all times, and his postural alignment made it even higher at all times. I worked with this seven-year-old baseball player for about 30 minutes, mostly discussing posture and setup position on the field and batting. He seemed to get it pretty well. We made an appointment for the next day. The next day his mom called me and said her son was 100 percent fine. I said, great, no problem. Give me a ring the next week and let me know how things were. She called the following week, said her son was completely pain free and feeling great.

Now I'm not looking to play hero in this situation. The kid's posture was awful, and it put a lot of wear on his spine. Making him aware of posture corrections off-loaded the problem and removed the causative factor for his pain. The reason it was so easy for this kid to become symptom free is because he didn't have twenty-plus years of bad posture in his muscle memory (like you do!) I said fix it and he did, just like that. But why did a seven-year-old have back pain for six months? Shouldn't the PE teacher have picked up something like this? Oh, wait—sorry, most state legislatures have made physical education, a class that should be focused on motor skills development, teamwork, and fun(!) into a "health" class that they have to sit down for or have eliminated it completely.

Yes—I'm going on a tangent here. But my hope is that some of you coaches and PE teachers reading this will rally and get things back on track again. I know budgets are tight, but you know what? It's about the kids, not $$$s. Kids in grade and high school should have integrated ACL injury prevention programs. You know what is really expensive? The bill for 100,000 ACL reconstructions that occur in the United States each year at $12,000-16,000 each. Did you know that ACL tears are seven to nine times more likely to occur in women? And did you know that ACL injury prevention programs are successful in decreasing injury rates? And did you also know that the exact same movement imbalances that cause the ACL to tear also cause patellofemoral pain syndrome, IT band pain, and medial tibial stress syndrome (shin splints). Every girl (and guy, too) in school should be able to describe step by step exactly how to tear your ACL, and show you exactly how they are correcting their mechanics to ensure they don't become a statistic. Movement skills. Developing a balanced muscle memory. Our system is set up to do nothing until people are broken. The fact that 82 percent of you are getting injured shows that the status quo is failing all of us. Let's put a dent in this statistic. Can one man move a mountain? No. But you could move your athletes' mechanics in the right direction and save them an injury. The interventional section has all the tools you'll need to begin. If you want more, look at the literature on ACL injury prevention, or go one step further and get a Sports-Metrics program going in your area. It's the right thing to do.

Conclusion

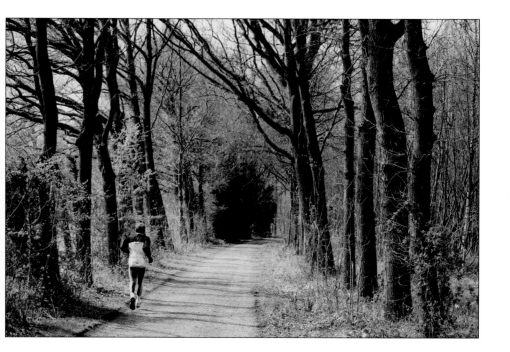

Where to Go from Here?

If you've made it this far, congratulations. You likely know more about running and how to perform specific tests and progressions to improve your running than most "experts." However, you are never done learning and exploring. Despite the well-referenced work I've included in this book, tomorrow you'll talk to your friend or mentor about this and they'll say "that's baloney—here's what I think!" Or maybe you'll read an article online on all the "Ten proposed benefits of stretching and why you need to do it this month!" It's fine to have opinions on many things. And since no two humans are exactly the same, it's even fine to adjust how you interpret advice if it works for you. However, it's not OK to spread the same old mantra that more miles are always better. It's not OK to think that rest will fix all your problems. It's not OK to think that more running will fix all your problems. It's not OK to think that every person on earth should run the same.

Specific interventions improve your parts. New skills help those parts work a system. More skills help the body deal with different paces, terrain, shoes, and competitive environments. The impetus here is on you. Maybe it's time we said, ask not what running can do for you, but what you can do for your running!

On the following pages, you'll find a number of references should you feel the need to look up more information on a particular topic. Heavy reading? Yes, it is. But we live in a world where the media reads a research abstract, takes one line out of it and spins it to fit their needs. If you want the truth, it's out there. You just have to go looking for it. And use that knowledge for the greater good—your good.

Great athletes come to the starting line prepared. They know what they've done. They've battled in the trenches. And they have a clear goal in focus that they strive for every day. Then they hit that goal and establish another. If you can keep pushing the limits, you keep the stakes alive in the big game of life. There's a great quote from Alan Webb, immediately after he broke Steve Scott's long-standing American mile record. He said, *"Thanks for setting the bar—you made me reach for something I didn't think I could do."* And to that, ladies and gentlemen, I'll leave you with one final question: How high is your bar?

Appendix A

Gait Vocabulary

The examination of running gait should begin with a little background on vocabulary. The term *gait cycle* is used to describe the parameters that occur in both walking and running. These parameters can be further broken down to define when, how long, and how rapidly the individual is in contact with the ground: *stride time, step time, stride length, gait velocity, and cadence.* Stride time is the time between contact of one foot to contact of the same foot. Step time refers to the period between contact of one foot to contact of the opposite foot. Stride length is the distance covered between contact of one foot to contact of the same foot, while step time reflects the distance from contact of one limb to the contact of the opposite limb. Gait velocity is distance covered over a set time. This is calculated as stride length divided by stride time and typically expressed as meters per second or miles per hour. Cadence refers to the number of steps taken in the course of a time, usually expressed as steps per minute. *Stance* refers to the foot on the ground, and *swing* refers to the leg swinging through the air.

Obviously, walking and running are different. Walking has periods of double support (both feet in contact with the ground at the same time) and single-leg support. Typically a walker spends 60 percent of his time in stance and 40 percent in swing during comfortable paces. These percentages can shift as walking speed increases; however, the key distinction of walking is that the person maintains one foot in contact with the ground at all times. Given that the world record for race walking a 10K is under 40 minutes, it is possible to move quite fast while subscribing to these guidelines. When walking, the body's center of mass oscillates slightly up and down such that the maximum forces experienced on one leg are never higher than 1.1 times the body weight. The long stance times and low forces during walking likely explains why we don't see catastrophic walking injuries.

By definition, running exists when the individual has periods of single leg support or flight. No double support can be seen in running. Runners spend approximately 30-40 percent of their time in stance (single-leg support) and 60-70 percent in swing (flight). During the flight phase, the body follows a parabolic curve similar to any projectile moving through the air. The increased rise and fall of the center of mass in distance running produces vertical forces approximately 2.2-2.7 times bodyweight. Sprinters generate forces as high as 3-3.1 times the bodyweight. The combination of short contact times, high forces, and repetition place great demands on the runner's tissues.

As running speed increases, the time spent in stance decreases, the time spent in swing increases, and a flight phase emerges. The only way to run faster is to cover more ground per stride and perform quicker strides. Stride length is limited somewhat by leg length and more so by joint mobility and the athlete's ability to generate sufficient force to move the center of mass forward. Running specific strength is critical to maintain stride length.

Appendix B

Strengthening References

Mikkola, J., H. Rusko, A. Nummela, T. Pollari, and K. Häkkinen. "Concurrent Endurance and Explosive Type Strength Training Improves Neuromuscular and Anaerobic Characteristics In Young Distance Runners." *Int J Sports Med.* 2007 Jul; 28(7):602-11. Epub 2007 Mar 20.

Mikkola, J., V. Vesterinen, R. Taipale, B. Capostagno, K. Häkkinen, and A. Nummela. "Effect of Resistance Training Regimens on Treadmill Running and Neuromuscular Performance in Recreational Endurance Runners." *J Sports Sci.* 2011 Oct; 29(13):1359-71. Epub 2011 Aug 22.

Spurrs, RW, AJ Murphy, and ML Watsford. "The Effect Of Plyometric Training On Distance Running Performance." *Eur J Appl Physiol.* 2003 Mar; 89(1):1-7. Epub 2002 Dec 24.

Støren O., Helgerud J., Støa EM, Hoff J. "Maximal Strength Training Improves Running Economy in Distance Runners." *Med Sci Sports Exerc.* 2008 Jun; 40(6):1087-92.

Taipale, RS, J. Mikkola, A. Nummela, V. Vesterinen, B. Capostagno, S. Walker, D. Gitonga, WJ Kraemer, and K. Häkkinen. "Strength Training in Endurance Runners." *Int J Sports Med.* 2010 Jul; 31(7):468-76. Epub 2010 Apr 29.

Yamamoto, LM, RM Lopez, JF Klau, DJ Casa, WJ Kraemer, and CM Maresh. "The Effects of Resistance Training on Endurance Distance Running Performance Among Highly Trained Runners: A Systematic Review." *J Strength Cond Res.* 2008 Nov; 22(6):2036-44.

Appendix C

Shoe References

Foot and Ankle Update. *In Proceedings of Healthsouth Educational Program.* Charlottesville, VA, 2002.

Running Course. *In Proceedings of Healthsouth Educational Program.* Charlottesville, VA, 2002.

Arroll, B., et al. "Patellofemoral Pain Syndrome. A Critical Review of the Clinical Trials On Nonoperative Therapy." *Am J Sports Med.* (25): 207-12, 1997.

Ball, KA, and M.J. Afheldt. "Evolution Of Foot Orthotics—Part 1: Coherent Theory Or Coherent Practice?" *J Manipulative Physiol Ther.* (25): 116-24, 2002.

Ball, KA, and M.J. Afheldt. "Evolution of Foot Orthotics—Part 2: Research Reshapes Long-standing Theory." *J Manipulative Physiol Ther.* (25): 125-34, 2002.

Barnes, RA, and PD Smith. "The Role of Footwear In Minimizing Lower Limb Injury." *J Sports Sci.* 12: 341-53, 1994.

Barrett, JR, et al. "High- versus Low-Top Shoes for the Prevention of Ankle Sprains In Basketball Players. A Prospective Randomized Study." *Am J Sports Med.* (21): 582-5, 1993.

Barton, CJ, et al. "The Efficacy of Foot Orthoses In the Treatment of Individuals with Patellofemoral Pain Syndrome: A Systematic Review." *Sports Med.* (40): 377-95, 2002.

Benard, M., et al. "Prescription Custom Foot Orthoses Practice Guidelines." *The American College of Foot and Ankle Orthopedics & Medicine.* 1-32, Bethesda, MD, 2004.

Bishop, M., et al. "Athletic Footwear, Leg Stiffness, and Running Kinematics." *J Athl Train.* (41): 387-92, 2006.

Bowring, B., and N. Chockalingam. "Conservative Treatment of Tibialis Posterior Tendon Dysfunction—A Review." *Foot (Edinb).* (20): 18-26, 2010.

Burns, J., et al. "Interventions for the Prevention and Treatment of Pes Cavus." *Cochrane Database Syst Rev.* CD006154, 2007.

Churchill, RS, and BG Donley. "Managing Injuries of the Great Toe." *Phys Sportsmed.* (26): 29-39, 1998.

Clarke, TE, EC Frederick, and CL Hamill. "The Effects of Shoe Design Parameters On Rearfoot Control In Running." *Med Sci Sports Exerc.* (15): 376-81, 1983.

Clinghan, R., et al. "Do You Get Value For Money When You Buy an Expensive Pair of Running Shoes?" *Br J Sports Med.* (42): 189-93, 2008.

Cornwall, M., and T. McPoil. "The Foot and Ankle: Current Concepts in Mechanics, Examination, and Orthotic Intervention." In: *Proceedings of Annual*

Conference & Exposition of the American Physical Therapy Association. Washington DC, 2003.

Cummings, GS, and EJ Higbie. "A Weight Bearing Method For Determining Forefoot Posting For Orthotic Fabrication." *Physiother Res Int.* (2): 42-50, 1997.

Dananberg, HJ, and M. Guiliano. "Chronic Low-Back Pain and Its Response to Custom-Made Foot Orthoses." *J Am Podiatr Med Assoc.* (89): 109-17, 1999.

Davis, IS, RA Zifchock, and AT Deleo. "A Comparison of Rearfoot Motion Control and Comfort Between Custom and Semicustom Foot Orthotic Devices." *J Am Podiatr Med Assoc.* (98): 394-403, 2008.

De Wit, B., D. De Clercq, and P. Aerts. "Biomechanical Analysis of the Stance Phase During Barefoot and Shod Running." *Journal of Biomechanics.* (33): 269-278, 2000.

Dicharry, JM. "Barefoot Running: Is Barefoot Better?" UVA Running Medicine Conference. Charlottesville, VA, 2010.

Dicharry, JM, et al. "Differences In Static and Dynamic Measures In Evaluation of Talonavicular Mobility In Gait." *J Orthop Sports Phys Ther.* (39): 628-34, 2009.

Dicharry, JM, et al. "Feed-Forward Foot Control In Running Gait." Poster presentation, GCMAS 2009.

Dixon, SJ, and DG Kerwin. "The Influence Of Heal(Sic) Lift Manipulation On Sagittal Plane Kinematics In Running." *Journal of Applied Biomechanics.* (15): 139-151, 1999.

Donatelli, RA, et al. "Biomechanical Foot Orthotics: A Retrospective Study." *J Orthop Sports Phys Ther.* (10): 205-12, 1988.

Ekenman, I., et al. "The Role of Biomechanical Shoe Orthoses In Tibial Stress Fracture Prevention." *Am J Sports Med.* (30): 866-70, 2002.

Finestone, A., et al. "Prevention of Stress Fractures Using Custom Biomechanical Shoe Orthoses." *Clin Orthop Relat Res.*182-90, 1999.

Genova, JM, and MT Gross. "Effect of Foot Orthotics On Calcaneal Eversion During Standing and Treadmill Walking For Subjects with Abnormal Pronation." *J Orthop Sports Phys Ther.* (30): 664-75, 2000.

Gross, ML, LB Davlin, and PM Evanski. "Effectiveness Of Orthotic Shoe Inserts In the Long-Distance Runner." *Am J Sports Med.* (19): 409-12, 1991.

Guldemond, NA, et al. "Casting Methods and Plantar Pressure: Effects Of Custom-Made Foot Orthoses On Dynamic Plantar Pressure Distribution." *J Am Podiatr Med Assoc.* (96): 9-18, 2006.

Handoll, HH, et al. "Interventions For Preventing Ankle Ligament Injuries." *Cochrane Database Syst Rev.* CD000018, 2001.

Hardin, EC, AJ van den Bogert, and J. Hamill. "Kinematic Adaptations During Running: Effects of Footwear, Surface, and Duration." *Med Sci Sports Exerc.* (36): 838-44, 2004.

Hawke, F., et al. "Custom-Made Foot Orthoses For the Treatment of Foot Pain." *Cochrane Database Syst Rev.* CD006801, 2008.

Heiderscheit BC, et al. "Effects of Step Rate Manipulation On Joint Mechanics During Running." *Medicine and Science in Sports and Exercise,* (43): 296-302, 2011.

Heiderscheit, B., J. Hamill, and D. Tiberio. "A Biomechanical Perspective: Do Foot Orthoses Work?" *Br J Sports Med.* (35): 4-5, 2001.

Hennig, EM, and TL Milani. "Pressure Distribution Measurements For Evaluation of Running Shoe Properties." *Sportverletz Sportschaden.* (14): 90-7, 2000.

Hume, P., et al. "Effectiveness of Foot Orthoses For Treatment and Prevention of Lower Limb Injuries : A Review." *Sports Med.* (38): 759-79, 2008.

Hryvniak, D., JM Dicharry, R. Wilder. "A Survery of Barefoot Running Injuries." Poster Presentation, UVA Running Medicine, 2012.

Hurley, MV. "The Role of Muscle Weakness In the Pathogenesis of Osteoarthritis." *Rheum Dis Clin North Am.* (25): 283-98, vi, 1999.

James, SL, BT Bates, and LR Osternig. "Injuries to Runners." *Am J Sports Med.* (6): 40-50, 1978.

Jarvinen, TA, et al. "Achilles Tendon Disorders: Etiology and Epidemiology." *Foot Ankle Clin.* (10): 255-66, 2005.

Kannus, P., and S. Niittymaki. "Which Factors Predict Outcome In the Nonoperative Treatment of Patellofemoral Pain Syndrome? A Prospective Follow-Up Study." *Med Sci Sports Exerc.* (26): 289-96, 1994.

Kerrigan, DC, et al. "The Effect of Running Shoes on Lower Extremity Joint Torques." *PM & R: The Journal Of Injury, Function, and Rehabilitation.* (1): 1058-1063, 2009.

Kitaoka, H.B., et al. "Effect of Foot Orthoses On 3-Dimensional Kinematics of Flatfoot: A Cadaveric Study." *Arch Phys Med Rehabil.* (83): 876-9, 2002.

Kong, PW, NG Candelaria, and DR Smith. "Running In New and Worn Shoes: A Comparison of Three Types of Cushioning Footwear." *Br J Sports Med.* (43): 745-9, 2009.

Kurz, MJ, and N. Stergiou. "The Spanning Set Indicates That Variability During the Stance Period of Running Is Affected by Footwear." *Gait Posture.* (17): 132-5, 2003.

Landorf, KB, and AM Keenan. "Efficacy of Foot Orthoses. What Does the Literature Tell Us?" *J Am Podiatr Med Assoc.* (90): 149-58, 2000.

Laughton, C., I. McClay Davis, and DS Williams. "A Comparison of Four Methods of Obtaining a Negative Impression of the Foot." *J Am Podiatr Med Assoc.* (92): 261-8, 2002.

Lee, SY, P. McKeon, and J. Hertel. "Does the Use of Orthoses Improve Self-Reported Pain and Function Measures In Patients with Plantar Fasciitis? A Meta-Analysis." *Phys Ther Sport.* (10): 12-8, 2009.

Lieberman, DE, et al. "Foot Strike Patterns and Collision Forces In Habitually Barefoot Versus Shod Runners." *Nature.* (463): 531-5, 2010.

Logan, S., et al. "Ground Reaction Force Differences Between Running Shoes, Racing Flats, and Distance Spikes In Runners." *Journal of Sports Science & Medicine.* (9): 147-153, 2010.

MacLean, CL. "Custom Foot Orthoses For Running." *Clin Podiatr Med Surg.* (18): 217-24, 2001.

MacLean, CL, IS Davis, and J. Hamill. "Short- and Long-Term Influences of a Custom Foot Orthotic Intervention On Lower Extremity Dynamics." *Clin Sport Med.* (18): 338-43, 2008.

McCaw, ST, ME Heil, and J. Hamill. "The Effect of Comments About Shoe Construction On Impact Forces During Walking." *Med Sci Sports Exerc.* (32): 1258-64, 2000.

Milgrom, C., et al. "The Effect of Shoe Sole Composition on In Vivo Tibial Strains During Walking." *Foot Ankle Int.* (22): 598-602, 2001.

Murley, GS, et al. "Effect of Foot Posture, Foot Orthoses and Footwear On Lower Limb Muscle Activity During Walking and Running: A Systematic Review." *Gait Posture.* (29): 172-87, 2009.

Nawoczenski, DA. "Nonoperative and Operative Intervention For Hallux Rigidus." *J Orthop Sports Phys Ther.* (29): 727-35, 1999.

Nawoczenski, DA, TM Cook, and CL Saltzman. "The Effect of Foot Orthotics on Three-Dimensional Kinematics of the Leg and Rearfoot During Running." *J Orthop Sports Phys Ther.* (21): 317-27, 1995.

Nigg, BM. "The Role of Impact Forces and Foot Pronation: A New Paradigm." *Clin J Sport Med.* (11): 2-9, 2001.

Nigg, BM, MA Nurse, and DJ Stefanyshyn. "Shoe Inserts and Orthotics For Sport and Physical Activities." *Med Sci Sports Exerc.* (31): S421-8, 1999.

Nigg, BM, et al. "The Effect of Material Characteristics of Shoe Soles on Muscle Activation and Energy Aspects During Running." *J Biomech.* (36): 569-75, 2003.

Nigg, BM, et al. "Effect of Shoe Inserts on Kinematics, Center of Pressure, and Leg Joint Moments During Running." *Med Sci Sports Exerc.* (35): 314-9, 2003.

Noll, KH. "The Use of Orthotic Devices In Adult Acquired Flatfoot Deformity." *Foot Ankle Clin.* (6): 25-36, 2001.

O'Connor, FG, RP Wilder, and R. Nirschl. *Textbook of Running Medicine.* New York; United States: McGraw-Hill, Medical Pub. Division, 2001.

Ogon, M., et al. "Footwear Affects the Behavior of Low Back Muscles When Jogging." *Int J Sports Med.* (22): 414-9, 2001.

Payne, C., and V. Chuter. "The Clash Between Theory and Science on the Kinematic Effectiveness of Foot Orthoses." *Clin Podiatr Med Surg.* (18): 705-13, vi, 2001.

Pratt, DJ. "A Critical Review of the Literature on Foot Orthoses." *J Am Podiatr Med Assoc.* (90): 339-41, 2000.

Razeghi, M., and ME Batt. "Biomechanical Analysis of the Effect of Orthotic Shoe Inserts: A Review of the Literature." *Sports Med.* (29): 425-38, 2000.

Reinschmidt, C., and BM Nigg. "Influence of Heel Height on Ankle Joint Moments In Running." *Med Sci Sports Exerc.* (27): 410-6, 1995.

Reinschmidt, C., and BM Nigg. "Current Issues in the Design of Running and Court Shoes." *Sportverletz Sportschaden.* (14): 71-81, 2000.

Richards, CE, PJ Magin, and R. Callister. "Is Your Prescription of Distance Running Shoes Evidence-Based?" *Br J Sports Med.* (43): 159-62, 2009.

Richie, DH, Jr. "Effects of Foot Orthoses on Patients with Chronic Ankle Instability." *J Am Podiatr Med Assoc.* (97): 19-30, 2007.

Robbins, S., and E. Waked. "Factors Associated with Ankle Injuries. Preventive Measures." *Sports Med.* (25): 63-72, 1998.

Roberts, ME, and CE Gordon. "Orthopedic Footwear. Custom-Made and Commercially Manufactured Footwear." *Foot Ankle Clin.* (6): 243-7, 2001.

Rome, K., HH Handoll, and R. Ashford. "Interventions For Preventing and Treating Stress Fractures and Stress Reactions of Bone of the Lower Limbs In Young Adults." *Cochrane Database Syst Rev.* CD000450, 2005.

Roy, JP, and DJ Stefanyshyn. "Shoe Midsole Longitudinal Bending Stiffness and Running Economy, Joint Energy, and EMG." *Med Sci Sports Exerc.* (38): 562-9, 2006.

Ryan, MB, et al. "The Effect of Three Different Levels of Footwear Stability on Pain Outcomes In Women Runners: A Randomised Control Trial." *Br J Sports Med,* 2009.

Sahrmann, S. *Diagnosis and Treatment of Movement Impairment Syndromes.* St. Louis, Mo. United States: Mosby, 2002.

Sekizawa, K., et al. "Effects of Shoe Sole Thickness on Joint Position Sense." *Gait Posture.* (13): 221-8, 2001.

Sharkey, NA, et al. "Strain and Loading of the Second Metatarsal During Heel-Lift." *J Bone Joint Surg Am.* (77): 1050-7, 1995.

Slemenda, C., et al. "Quadriceps Weakness and Osteoarthritis of the Knee." *Ann Intern Med.* (127): 97-104, 1997.

Squadrone, R., and C. Gallozzi. "Biomechanical and Physiological Comparison of Barefoot and Two Shod Conditions In Experienced Barefoot Runners." *Journal of Sports Medicine and Physical Fitness.* (49): 6-13, 2009.

Stacoff, A., X. Kalin, and E. Stussi. "The Effects of Shoes on the Torsion and Reafoot Motion In Running." *Medicine and Science in Sports and Exercise.* (23): 482-490, 1991.

Stefanyshyn, DJ, and BM Nigg. "Energy Aspects Associated with Sport Shoes." *Sportverletz Sportschaden.* (14): 82-9, 2000.

Appendix D

Gait References

Biewener, AA, et al. "Muscle Mechanical Advantage of Human Walking and Running: Implications For Energy Cost." *J Appl Physiol.* 97(6): 2266-74, 2004.

Birrer, RB, et al. "Biomechanics of Running." In: O'Conor F., Wilder R. (eds). *The Textbook of Running Medicine.* New York: McGraw Hill, 2001, p. 11-19.

Cavanagh PR, and MA Lafortune. "Ground Reaction Forces In Distance Running." *J Biomech.* (13): 397-406, 1980.

Chang, Y., et al. "The Independent Effects of Gravity and Inertia on Running Mechanics." *J Exp Bio.* (203): 229-238, 2000.

Chumanov, ES, BC Heiderscheit, and DG Thelen. "The Effect of Speed and Influence of Individual Muscles on Hamstring Mechanics During the Swing Phase of Sprinting." *J Biomech.* 40(16): 3555-62, 2007.

Della Croce, U., A. Cappozzo, and DC Krrigan. "Pelvic and Lower Anatomical Landmark Calibration and Its Propagation to Bone Geometry and Joint Angles." *Med Biol Eng Comput* 37(2): 155-61, 1999.

Donelan, JM, R. Kram, and AD Kuo. "Mechanical Work For Step to Step Transitions Is a Major Determinant of the Metabolic Cost of Human Walking." *J Exp Bio.* (205): 3717-3727, 2002.

Donelan, JM, R. Kram, and AD Kuo. "Simultaneous Positive and Negative External Mechanical Work In Human Walking." *J Biomech.* (35): 117-124, 2002.

Dicharry, JM. "Clinical Running Gait Analysis." In: O'Conor F., Wilder R. (eds). *Textbook of Running Medicine, 2nd Ed.* McGraw Hill, 2012.

Dicharry, JM. "Kinematics and Kinetics of Gait: From Lab to Clinic." *Clin Sports Med.* 29(3): 347-64, 2010.

Dicharry, JM, et al. "Differences In Static and Dynamic Measures In Evaluation of Talonavicular Mobility In Gait." *J Orthop Sports Phys Ther.* 39(8): 628-34, 2009.

Drewes, LK, et al. "Dorsiflexion Deficit During Jogging with Chronic Ankle Instability." *Journal of Science and Medicine in Sport.* 12(6): 685-687, Nov. 2009.

Dugan, SA, and KP Bhat. "Biomechanics and Analysis of Running Gait." *Phys Med Rehabil Clin N Am.* 16(3): 603-21, Aug. 2005.

Farley, CT, and O. Gonzalez. "Leg Stiffness and Stride Frequency In Human Running." *J Biomech.* 29(2): 181-6, Feb. 1996.

Franz, JR, et al. "Changes In the Coordination of Hip and Pelvis Kinematics with Mode of Locomotion." *Gait Posture.* 29(3): 494-8, April 2009.

Frigo, C., et al. "Functionally Oriented and Clinically Feasible Quantitative Gait Analysis Method." *Med Biol Eng Comput.* 36(2): 179-185, 1998.

Gerlach, KE, et al. "Kinetic Changes with Fatigue and Relationship to Injury In Female Runners." *Med Sci Sports Exerc.* 37(4): 657-63, April 2005.

Giannini, S., et al. "Gait Analysis: Methodologies and Clinical Applications." BTS Bioengineering Technology and Systems. Amsterdam, Netherlands, 1994.

Gottschall, JS, and R. Kram. "Ground Reaction Forces During Downhill and Uphill Running." *J Biomech.* 38(3): 445-52, 2005.

Grindstaff, T., et al. "Neuromuscular Control Training Programs and Non-contact Anterior Cruciate Ligament Injury Rates in Female Athletes: A Numbers-Needed-to-Treat Analysis." *J Athl Train.* 41(4): 450–456, 2006.

Hart, JM, et al. "Jogging Gait Kinetics Following Fatiguing Lumbar Paraspinal Exercise." *J Electromyogr Kinesiol.* (6): e458-64. Epub 2008 Dec 16.

Heiderschiet, BC, et al. "Effects of Step Rate Manipulation on Joint Mechanics during Running." *Med Sci Sports Exerc.* June 23, 2010.

Hinrichs, RN. "Upper Extremity Function In Distance Running." In: Cavanaugh, PR (ed.) *Biomechanics of Distnce Running.* Champaign, IL: Human Kinetics, 1990, (4): 107-133.

Hodges, PW. "Core Stability Exercise In Chronic Low Back Pain." *Orthop Clin North Am.* 34(2): 245-54, 2003.

Hreljac, A., RN Marshall, and PA Hume. "Evaluation of Lower Extremity Overuse Injury Potential In Runners." Med Sci Sports Exerc. 32(9): 1635-41, 2000.

Hreljac, A. "Impact and Overuse Injuries In Runners." *Med Sci Sports Exerc.* 36(5): 845-9, 2004.

Jacobs, R., MF Bobbert, and GJ Van Ingen Schenau. "Mechanical Output from Individual Muscles During Explosive Leg Extensions: The Role of Biarticular Muscles." *J Biomech.* 29(4): 513-23, 1996.

Khan, Karim M., MD, et al. "Overuse Tendinosis, Not Tendinitis." *The Physician and Sportsmedicine.* 28(5), May 2000.

Kerdok, AE, et al. "Energetics and Mechanics of Human Running on Surfaces of Different Stiffnesses." *J Appl Physiol.* 92(2): 469-78, 2002.

Kerrigan, DC, and U. Della Croce. "Gait Analysis." In: O'Conner, FG, et al (eds): *Sports Medicine, Just the Facts.* McGraw-Hill: 2005, pp. 126-130.

Kerrigan, DC, et al. "The Effect of Running Shoes on Lower Extremity Joint Torques." *PM&R.* 1(12), Dec. 2009.

Kerrigan, DC, and JE Edelstein. "Gait." In: Gonzalez, EG, et al (eds): *The Physiological Basis of Rehabilitation Medicine.* Boston: Butterworth-Heineman, 2001, pp. 397-416.

Kram, R., and CR Taylor. "Energetics of Running: A New Perspective." *Nature.* 346(6281): 265-7, Jul 19, 1990.

Leardini, A., et al. "Rear-Foot, Mid-Foot, and Fore-Foot Motion During the Stance Phase of Gait." *Gait Posture.* (25): 453-462, 2007.

Leadnini, A., et al. "An Anatomical Based Protocol For the Description of Foot Segment Kinematics During Gait." *Clin Biomech.* (14): 528-536, 1999.

Leardini, A., et al. "Human Movement Analysis Using Stereophotogrammetry. Part 3: Soft Tissue Artifact Assessment and Compensation." *Gait Posture.* (21): 212-225, 2005.

Lieberman, DE, et al. "Foot Strike Patterns and Collision Forces In Habitually Barefoot Versus Shod Runners." *Nature.* (463): 531-5, 2010.

Mann, RA. "Biomechanics of Running." In: Nicholas, JA, and EB Hershman, editors. *The Lower Extremity and Spine in Sports Medicine, Vol. 1.* St Louis: The C.V. Mosby Company; 1986. p. 395–411.

Martin, PE, and DW Morgan. "Biomechanical Considerations For Economical Walking and Running." *Med Sci Sports Exer.* 24(4): 407-74, 1992.

McCann, DJ, and BK Higginson. "Training to Maximize Economy of Motion In Running Gait." *Curr. Sports Med. Rep.* 7(3): 158-162.

McKeon, P., and J. Hertel. "Systematic Review of Postural Control and Lateral Ankle Instability, Part II: Is Balance Training Clinically Effective." *J Athl Train.* 43(3): 305–315, 2008.

McPoil, T., and MW Cornwall. "Relationship Between Neutral Subtalar Joint Posiion and Pattern of Rearfoot Motion During Walking." *Foot Ankle Int.* (15): 141-145, 1994.

Nester, C. et al. "Foot Kinematics During Walking Measured Using Bone and Surface Mounted Markers." *J Biomech.* (40): 3412-3423, 2007.

Nigg, BM. "The Role of Impact Forces and Foot Pronation: A New Paradigm." *Clin J Sport Med.* 11(1): 2-9, 2001.

Noehren, B., J. Scholz, and I. Davis. "The Effect of Real-Time Gait Retraining on Hip Kinematics, Pain and Function In Subjects with Patellofemoral Pain Syndrome." *Br J Sports Med.* June 28, 2010.

Novacheck, TF. "The Biomechanics of Running." *Gait Posture.* (7): 77-95, 1998.

Novacheck, TF, JP Tros, and L. Schutte. *Running and Sprinting: A Dynamic Analysis* (video cd/rom) St. Paul MN, Gillette Children's Hospital, 1996.

O'Connor, JA, and LE Lanyon. "The Influence of Strain Rate on Adaptive Bone Remodeling." *J Biomechanics.* (15): 767-781, 1982.

Perry, J. *Gait Analysis: Normal and Pathological Function.* Thorofare, NJ: SLACK, 1992.

Pope, RP. "Prevention of Pelvic Stress Fractures In Female Army Recruits." *Mil Med.* 164(5): 370-3, 1999.

Prilutsky, BI, and VM Zatsiorsky. "Tendon Action of Two Joint Muscles: Transfer of Mechanical Energy Between Two Joints During Jumping, Landing, and Running." *J Biomech* 27(1): 25-34, 1994.

Provenzano, PP, et al. "Hindlimb Unloading Alters Ligament Healing." *J Appl Physiol.* (94): 314-324, 2003.

Richards, CE, PJ Magin, and R. Callister. "Is Your Prescription of Distance Running Shoes Evidence-Based?" *J Sports Med.* (43): 159-162, 2009.

Riley, PO, et al. "A Kinematics and Kinetic Comparison of Overground and Treadmill Running." *Med Sci Sports Exerc.* 40(6): 1093-100, 2008.

Roberts, et al. "Muscular Force in Running Turkeys: The Economy of Minimizing Work." *Science.* 275(5303): 1113-5, 1997.

Scott, SH, and DA Winter. "Internal Forces At Chronic Running Injury Sites." *Med Sci Sports Exerc.* (22): 357-369, 1999.

Squadrone, R., and C. Galozzo. March 2009. "Biomechanical and Physiological Comparison of Barefoot and Two Shod Conditions In Experienced Barefoot Runners." *J Sports Med Phys Fitness.* 49(1): 6-13.

Souza, RB, and CM Powers. "Differences In Hip Kinematics, Muscle Strength, and Muscle Activation Between Subjects with and Without Patellofemoral Pain." *J Orthop Sports Phys Ther.* 39(1): 12-9, 2009.

Souza, RB, and CM Powers. "Predictors of Hip Internal Rotation During Running: An Evaluation of Hip Strength and Femoral Structure In Women with and Without Patellofemoral Pain." *Am J Sports Med.* 37(3): 579-87, 2009.

Teunissen, L., A. Grabowski, and R. Kram. "The Effects of Independenly Altering Body Weight and Body Mass on the Metabolic Cost of Running." *J of Exp Bio.* (210): 4418-27, 2007.

Thelen, DG, et al. "Neuromusculoskeletal Models Provide Insights into the Mechanisms and Rehabilitation of Hamstring Strains." *Exerc Sport Sci Rev.* 34(3): 135-41, 2006.

Wright, S., and PS Weyland. "The Application of Ground Force Explains the Energetic Cost of Running Backward and Forward." *The Journal of Experimental Biology.* (204): 1805–1815, 2001.